The Stroke Center Handbook

The Stroke Center Handbook
Organizing Care for Better Outcomes
A Guide to Stroke Center Development and Operations

Marilyn M Rymer MD

Mid America Brain and Stroke Institute
Saint Luke's Hospital
Kansas City, MO, USA

Debbie Summers MSN

Mid America Brain and Stroke Institute
Saint Luke's Hospital
Kansas City, MO, USA

and

Pooja Khatri MD

Department of Neurology
University of Cincinnati
Cincinnati, OH, USA

With contributions from

Stephen J Page PhD FAHA
Director
Neuromotor Recovery and Rehabilitation Laboratory
Drake Rehabilitation Center
Cincinnati, OH, USA

Thomas A Tomsick MD
Director of Neuroradiology and Interventional Neuroradiology
Department of Radiology
University of Cincinnati Medical Center
Cincinnati, OH, USA

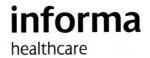

© 2007 Informa UK Ltd

First published in the United Kingdom in 2007 by Informa Healthcare Ltd, 4 Park Square,
Milton Park, Abingdon, Oxon OX14 4RN
Informa Healthcare is a trading division of Informa UK Ltd
Registered Office: 37/41 Mortimer Street, London W1T 3JH
Registered in England and Wales Number 1072954.

Tel: +44 (0)20 7017 6000
Fax: +44 (0)20 7017 6336
Email: info.medicine@tandf.co.uk
Website: www.informahealthcare.com

Although every effort has been made to ensure that all owners of copyright material have
been acknowledged in this publication, we would be glad to acknowledge in subsequent
reprints or editions any omissions brought to our attention.

Although every effort has been made to ensure that drug doses and other information are
presented accurately in this publication, the ultimate responsibility rests with the
prescribing physician. Neither the publishers nor the authors can be held responsible for
errors or for any consequences arising from the use of information contained herein. For
detailed prescribing information or instructions on the use of any product or procedure
discussed herein, please consult the prescribing information or instructional material issued
by the manufacturer.

A CIP record for this book is available from the British Library.
Library of Congress Cataloging-in-Publication Data

Data available on application

ISBN-10: 1 84214 286 0
ISBN-13: 978 1 84214 286 8

Distributed in North and South America by
Taylor & Francis
6000 Broken Sound Parkway, NW, (Suite 300)
Boca Raton, FL 33487, USA

Within Continental USA
Tel: 1 (800) 272 7737; Fax: 1 (800) 374 3401
Outside Continental USA
Tel: (561) 994 0555; Fax: (561) 361 6018
Email: orders@crcpress.com

Distributed in the rest of the world by
Thomson Publishing Services
Cheriton House
North Way
Andover, Hampshire SP10 5BE, UK
Tel: +44 (0)1264 332424
Email: tps.tandfsalesorder@thomson.com

Composition by Scribe Design Ltd, Ashford, Kent, UK
Printed and bound in India by Replika Press Pvt Ltd

Dedication

To the Stroke Team at Saint Luke's Mid America Brain and Stroke Institute and the University of Cincinnati.

Contents

Preface

The incidence and prevalence of stroke is increasing. Stroke is the second leading cause of death worldwide and the leading cause of adult disability. Treatment is available for acute intervention and there is accumulating evidence regarding prevention of complications, secondary prevention, and new approaches to rehabilitation. The time is right to design processes and infrastructure that will assure every stroke victim the best possible outcome.

The purpose of this book is to provide insight and information to physicians, nurses, therapists, and administrators who are planning the programs necessary to do this work, regardless of the size of the hospital or available workforce. The evidence directing therapy for stroke is changing rapidly. The recommendations for the management of stroke that are included are based on current evidence and future trends, but they will change as new data become available. The hope, however, is that the infrastructure and processes described in this book are foundations that will stand the test of time and assure standardization of care in stroke centers while providing the flexibility to incorporate new therapies as evidence evolves.

Providing good outcomes to stroke victims is time-dependent, labor intensive, and complicated. Nevertheless, it is the responsibility of every health care organization to have a plan in place to meet the challenge when the patient arrives at the door.

1

Setting the goal for the stroke center

The goal of the stroke center is to provide the best possible outcome for every patient. An organized approach to care can be achieved in every hospital, and the first issue to address in planning is to determine what level of care can be realistically provided.

The continuum of care for stroke can be divided into three distinct phases, each requiring different resources, personnel and infrastructure.

PHASE I: ACUTE STROKE TREATMENT

It is very likely that acute stroke treatment will always be time-dependent, with the best outcomes resulting from the earliest intervention.

Options for acute stroke treatment fall into two categories. The following examples have not all been proven effective but are meant to be illustrative.

Non-invasive treatment requires no surgical or interventional access.
• Intravenous (IV) thrombolytics/thrombin inhibitors
• Neuroprotective agents
• Agents to prevent hematoma enlargement
• Hypothermia
• Ultrasound enhanced thrombolysis.

Invasive treatment requires interventional or surgical access.
• Mechanical embolectomy
• Intra-arterial thrombolysis
• Aneurysm coiling or clipping
• Surgical clot removal.

Important questions to be addressed if acute stroke intervention is one of the goals:
1. Is time-dependent acute stroke intervention going to be offered 24/7?
2. Is non-invasive acute treatment going to be provided? (Checklist 1)
3. Is invasive acute treatment going to be provided? (Checklist 2)

If the answer to question no. 1 is NO and acute stroke treatment is not going to be available or only available during the day, then it is critical to have a plan for rapid transfer or bypass for patients who present within the treatment time window (Figure 1.1 and Chapter 3).

Figure 1.1

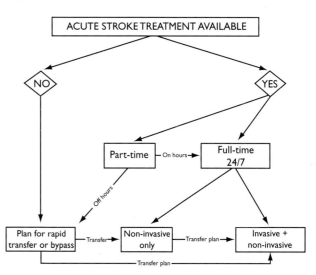

Algorithm for acute stroke treatment

1

Checklist 1: Resources required for non-invasive acute treatment

- Emergency department personnel trained to triage and diagnose acute stroke
- Physician trained in acute stroke treatment available 24/7
- Neuroimaging available to be done and interpreted in 30–45 minutes
- STAT lab
- Pharmacy to mix drug or drug available in Emergency Department
- Intensive care unit (ICU) or step-down unit for patient admission
- Stroke care path/flowchart
- Order set for stroke and for acute treatment selected.

Checklist 2: Additional resources required for invasive stroke treatment

- Interventional radiology or surgical team ready in 30 minutes
- Endovascular surgeon or neurosurgeon available 24/7
- Properly equipped surgical or interventional suite(s).

PHASE II: MEDICAL/SURGICAL MANAGEMENT

There is conclusive evidence that stroke victims, even those ineligible for acute intervention, who are managed in an organized stroke center have better outcomes and decreased mortality.[1] Care paths, standing order sets, and highly trained nurses make up the basic infrastructure that guarantees standardized care in five areas.

- Tight control of physiologic parameters (Chapter 6)
- Prevention of complications (Chapter 7)
- Diagnosis of the cause of the stroke (Chapter 8)
- Plan for secondary prevention (Chapter 8)
- Early rehabilitation (Chapter 9).

Should structural disease be diagnosed then surgical or interventional repair should be considered (Chapter 8).

Checklist 3: Resources to achieve best practice medical/surgical management of stroke

- Physicians knowledgeable in the diagnosis and management of stroke
- Stroke center nurses trained in neurological assessment and competent to use specialized monitoring equipment
- Staffing level to guarantee frequent neurological assessments and blood pressure (BP) monitoring by nurses
- Neuroimaging to include computed tomography (CT), magnetic resonance imaging (MRI), computerized tomographic angiography (CTA), magnetic resonance angiography (MRA), cerebral angiography
- Carotid artery imaging: ultrasound, CTA, MRA
- Echocardiography: 2D echo, transesophageal echo with protocol for diagnosis of atrial septal defect, patent foramen ovale (PFO), atrial septal aneurysm (ASA)
- Care paths for ischemic and hemorrhagic stroke and transient ischemic attack (TIA) to address acute and subacute management, prevention of complications, secondary prevention and early rehabilitation (Appendix)
- Standing order sets for stroke, stroke intervention, and TIA (Appendix)
- Designated stroke center beds.

PHASE III: REHABILITATION

It is clear that early access to rehabilitation specialists improves outcomes and decreases length of stay on the acute hospital unit. The goal would be to have evaluations by physical, occupational, and speech therapy on day 1 and initiation of plans for the next phase of rehabilitation should it be needed.

Checklist 4: Rehabilitation services available

- Physical therapy
- Occupational therapy
- Speech therapy
- Inpatient rehabilitation unit.

If the patient is transferred to the inpatient rehabilitation unit, the care path from the stroke center can coordinate with the care path on the rehabilitation unit.

Once the analysis of the level of care that can be realistically provided for the three phases of care is complete, then the pertinent sections of this handbook can be used to guide the stroke center's development. Ideally, hospitals capable of delivering primary care will establish relationships with tertiary care institutions to carry out the more sophisticated and resource-intense interventions and evaluations.

In the US, the Brain Attack Coalition has published Recommendations for the Components of a Primary Stroke Center[2] and of a Comprehensive Stroke Center.[3]

MAJOR COMPONENTS OF A PRIMARY STROKE CENTER

Patient care areas:
- Acute stroke teams
- Written care protocols
- Emergency medical services
- Emergency department
- Stroke units in hospitals planning to admit stroke patients
- Neurosurgical services.

Support services:
- Commitment and support of medical organization; a stroke center director
- Neuroimaging services
- Laboratory services
- Outcome and quality improvement activities
- Continuing medical education.

MAJOR COMPONENTS OF A COMPREHENSIVE STROKE CENTER

Personnel with expertise in the following areas:
- Vascular neurology
- Vascular neurosurgery
- Advanced practice nurse
- Vascular surgery
- Diagnostic radiology/neuroradiology
- Interventional/endovascular physicians
- Critical care medicine
- Physical medicine and rehabilitation
- Rehabilitation therapy (physical, occupational, speech therapy)
- Staff stroke nurse(s)
- Swallowing assessment.

Diagnostic techniques:
- MRI with diffusion
- MRA/magnetic resonance venography (MRV)
- CTA
- Digital cerebral angiography
- Transcranial doppler (TCD)
- Carotid duplex ultrasound
- Transesophageal echocardiography (TEE).

Surgical and interventional therapies:
- Carotid endarterectomy
- Clipping of intracranial aneurysm
- Placement of ventriculostomy
- Hematoma removal/draining
- Placement of intracranial pressure transducer
- Endovascular ablation of aneurysms/arteriovenous malformations (AVMs)
- Intra-arterial reperfusion therapy
- Endovascular treatment of vasospasm.

Infrastructure:
- Stroke unit
- ICU
- Operating room staffed 24/7
- Interventional services coverage 24/7
- Stroke registry.

Educational/research programs:
- Community education
- Community prevention
- Professional education
- Patient education.

Leadership is critical to the successful integration of these components into a finely tuned stroke treatment system. The Brain Attack Coalition (BAC) recommends there be a physician and nurse director for the program and strong relationships with the Emergency Department and emergency medical services (EMS) providers.

The Joint Commission on the Accreditation of Hospitals Organization (JCAHO) Disease Specific Certification in Stroke is based on having the Primary Stroke Center components in place as well as the ability to monitor some or all of the following performance measures:

- Deep vein thrombosis prophylaxis
- Discharged on antithrombotics
- Patients with atrial fibrillation receiving anticoagulation therapy
- Tissue plasminogen activator considered
- Antithrombotic medication within 48 hours of hospitalization
- Screen for dysphagia
- Stroke education

- Smoking cessation
- A plan for rehabilitation was considered.

Once the planning team has determined the level of service to be provided then setting yearly goals for the stroke center helps focus energy and provides a basis for measuring success.

Categories of goals:

- Performance measures
  - Clinical: case volume, mortality rate, disposition, length of stay, acute intervention rate, complication rate
  - Financial: product line contribution margin, cost per case
  - Patient and family satisfaction
- Educational programs and stroke screenings: public, professional
- Research
- Infrastructure and personnel
- Marketing.

Questions to consider while setting the goal for the stroke center

1. What kind of stroke services will be provided?

2. What is the feasibility of success and acceptance of the stroke program?
3. What are the opportunities and barriers?
4. Who will be the core team members? Who do we already have and who do we need to recruit?
5. What will it take to get buy-in from key constituents: neurologists, neurosurgeons, radiologists, administrators, primary care physicians, board members?
6. Who should be on the planning team?
7. What will the budget be?
8. How will we communicate what we are doing?

REFERENCES

1. Collaborative systematic review of the randomised trials of organised inpatient (stroke unit) care after stroke. Stroke Unit Trialists' Collaboration. BMJ 1997; 314: 1151–9.
2. Alberts HJ, Hademenos G, Latchaw RE et al. Recommendations for the establishment of primary stroke centers. Brain Attach Coalition. JAMA 2000; 283(23): 3102–8.
3. Alberts HJ, Latchaw RE, Selman WR et al. Recommendations for comprehensive stroke centers: a consensus statement from the Brain Attack Coalition. Stroke 2005; 36: 1597–618.

2

Stroke center organization

By the very nature of the disease, stroke care requires coordination of multiple clinical services. This chapter addresses the components of a comprehensive stroke program that would include research and education as well as the core clinical work. Smaller centers can adapt this structure to their resources, personnel and goals.

For the stroke center to be successful, it must have strong leadership and be backed up by organizational will. The strongest stroke centers are led by an administrator committed to the success of the program and a physician and nurse champion. Taking excellent care of patients with strokes requires cooperation from multiple hospital departments and dedicated clinicians. An effective partner in administration is important to the success of the clinicians. It is also important to develop a written vision, mission, and strategic/business plan for the stroke center early in the process of organization and to gain support for that vision and plan from the highest levels of responsibility in the organization, the board

of trustees, and senior hospital administration. These written documents will vary in complexity with the size of the program, but even a basic plan serves as a guide for the work of the stroke center. Yearly review of the documents provides an opportunity to evaluate progress and set goals for the future (Box 2.1). A board member or committee of the board that serves as a liaison from the stroke center leaders to the board of the hospital and to the community can be very important to the successful launch and maintenance of the stroke program.

THE PEOPLE

Core leadership team

Designating a medical director, nurse coordinator, and administrator for the stroke program sets up lines of responsibility for program development and clinical quality. In the most basic programs these responsibilities may be as simple as developing the policy and mechanism for transfer of acute stroke patients to a center capable of acute intervention and standards of care for those patients not eligible for transfer. The job descriptions that follow are typical for tertiary care community hospital stroke centers, but can be easily adapted to less complex programs or to academic programs where there may be neurology residents or stroke fellows.

Medical director

The medical director is often a neurologist, but this is not a requirement. A physician with interest and expertise in the care of stroke patients is all that is needed. In larger programs this position is generally

---

Box 2.1 Stroke program

Stroke program vision: The stroke program will provide the best possible outcome for every patient.

Stroke program mission: The mission of the stroke program is to decrease the incidence and morbidity from stroke in the region through clinical excellence, research and education.

Stroke program plan:
1. Stroke team leadership and personnel
2. Stroke center location
3. Clinical tools
4. Budget
5. Policies

financially compensated by the hospital based on the time commitment. The role of the medical director is to provide leadership in planning, clinical quality, communication, research, and fund raising. The job description may include:

- Develop vision, mission, and strategic plan for the stroke center
- Set and review yearly goals (Chapter 1)
- Communicate information regarding the stroke program to the hospital board, administration, medical staff, laboratory, pharmacy, radiology and emergency departments, marketing, emergency medical service (EMS) providers, lay community supporters, and outlying community medical personnel
- Assure clinical quality by developing standardized protocols and order sets as well as conducting regular case reviews
- Continually review current evidence regarding stroke prevention, diagnosis, treatment, and rehabilitation
- Lead development of stroke database and stroke research program
- Review clinical and cost outcome data on a regular basis
- Assist in development of educational programs for professional staff and the community
- Develop philanthropic support for the stroke program
- Publish in peer-reviewed journals and present data at local and national meetings
- Write an annual report for the stroke program.

Nurse coordinator

The role of the nurse coordinator is essential regardless of the size or complexity of the stroke program. In some programs this may be an advanced practice nurse (APN) who can do independent patient assessment and billing, but in most settings the nurse coordinator is a hospital employee with expertise in neuroscience. Depending on the size of the program, the role of stroke team coordinator may be combined with other related responsibilities. The nurse coordinator works closely with the medical director and shares responsibility for stroke center operations. The job description may include:

- Set and review yearly goals for the stroke program

- Lead development of care paths, protocols and standing order sets for ischemic and hemorrhagic stroke, transient ischemic attack (TIA), etc. and update yearly based on current evidence
- Provide education for nurses in all locations of the hospital who are taking care of patients with strokes, including instruction aimed at NIH Stroke Scale (NIHSS) certification (Appendix)
- Review clinical quality using case reviews for stroke center nurses
- Support entry of information into the stroke database
- Support stroke clinical research
- Provide education to EMS providers, emergency room staff in referring hospitals, and members of the community
- If trained to an APN level, provide first response to acute stroke calls.

Stroke program administrator

In larger programs, the administrator for the stroke center may be a full-time position. However, in many hospitals this assignment may be combined with other related responsibilities. Job description may include:

- Strategically plan with the stroke team clinicians to anticipate equipment and personnel needs
- Set and review yearly goals for the stroke program
- Represent the stroke center at administrative and budget meetings
- Build hospital processes that support the clinical and research activities of the stroke team
- Provide space and supplies for the stroke team
- Supervise the members of the stroke team who are hospital employees.

The three roles described above bridge the activities of the stroke teams and the rest of the stroke program operations (Figure 2.1).

The clinical team

The composition of the clinical team will vary depending on what level of service is to be provided. If all phases of clinical services for stroke are to be offered, then it is ideal to have neurologists, neurosurgeons, interventional radiologists, emergency

Figure 2.1

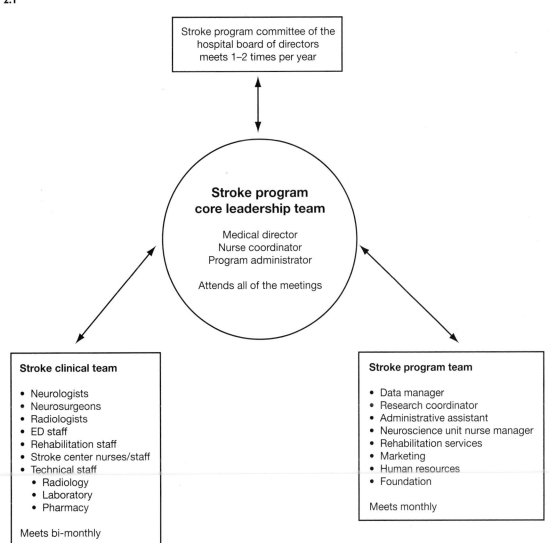

Stroke program committee of the
hospital board of directors
meets 1–2 times per year

**Stroke program
core leadership team**

Medical director
Nurse coordinator
Program administrator

Attends all of the meetings

Stroke clinical team

- Neurologists
- Neurosurgeons
- Radiologists
- ED staff
- Rehabilitation staff
- Stroke center nurses/staff
- Technical staff
  - Radiology
  - Laboratory
  - Pharmacy

Meets bi-monthly

Stroke program team

- Data manager
- Research coordinator
- Administrative assistant
- Neuroscience unit nurse manager
- Rehabilitation services
- Marketing
- Human resources
- Foundation

Meets monthly

Stroke teams: composition and communication

department (ED) staff, rehabilitation physicians, nurses and therapists, stroke center nurses and technical support staff in radiology, lab and pharmacy represented on the team. Some members of this team will need to be available 24/7. Programs may choose to use hospitalists, intensivists, emergency medicine or primary care physicians in the role of the stroke neurologist. The ED, radiology, lab, and pharmacy may find it beneficial to designate one person who is the principal communication link to the stroke team.

The responsibilities of the clinical team are to take excellent care of the patient to ensure the best possible outcome and to communicate with the family and referring physicians. The members of the team will change depending on where the patient is and what care is being provided. For each of the follow-ing phases of care a list of team members should be developed:

- Acute intervention in the ED, radiology suite or operating room
- Post intervention management in the intensive care unit (ICU) or step down unit
- Prevention of complications, evaluation of cause of the stroke and plan for secondary prevention in the acute care stroke center
- Rehabilitation in the rehabilitation department or units.

The expertise of the nurses involved in the care of stroke patients is one of the critical success factors for an outstanding stroke program. Nurses in the ED,

ICU, and acute stroke center should have organized stroke education and be certified to use the NIHSS (Appendix).

Stroke program team

Additional team members can enrich and support the activities of the stroke program. Some of these people work primarily to support the stroke program and some function in a liaison role to connect the stroke team with other resources and departments of the hospital.

Data manager

Tracking clinical and financial data is critically important in operating an efficient and high-quality stroke program. Administrative data may be used for an overview of mortality, disposition, complications, and costs. Using a stroke-specific database gives much more detailed information and is useful for clinical analyses, trending, benchmarking, and research. Several commercial stroke databases are available or one can be developed that is unique to the institution (Box 2.2). The nurse coordinator may be able to manage the data, but most larger programs have a dedicated position for this work. Job description may include:

- Choose the most appropriate database or develop one
- Enter data for all stroke admissions
- Determine what outcome measures will be tracked: e.g. mortality, complications, disposition, 90-day function (mRankin)
- Develop process for obtaining 90-day outcome data
- Coordinate with administrative and financial datasets to avoid duplication of effort
- Produce regular reports tracking volume, outcomes, and performance measures
- Provide data to support clinical and research operations.

Research coordinator

The opportunities for stroke centers to participate in clinical research continue to grow. Clinical trials can be successfully run in community hospitals as well as academic centers, and are often a source of excitement and pride for the team. The research coordinator is generally a nurse experienced in the care of stroke patients. A good clinical nurse can be trained to understand the regulatory requirements and other aspects of directing a research trial. Formal courses are available for in-depth training and some coordinators may choose to become formally certified (Box 2.3). After the research program is up and running, the salary for the coordinator can be paid out of income from the studies. In some programs, the nurse coordinator for the stroke team may also be the research coordinator. If the clinical trial involves acute stroke management or intervention, then the question of 24/7 coverage has to be addressed. Job description may include:

- Obtain training in all aspects of clinical research
- Submit research protocols to the Institutional Review Board (IRB) and comply with all IRB rules
- Develop the research budget
- Coordinate and train all participating departments and personnel
- Develop standing order sets for trials
- Develop checklists of inclusion/exclusion criteria to aid clinicians in enrolling appropriate subjects
- Consent and enroll subjects
- Submit timely case report forms
- Meet with study monitors
- Attend investigator meetings.

Box 2.2 Stroke Databases

Coverdell Registry, CDC
http://www.cdc.gov/cvh/stroke_registry.htm

Get With the Guidelines, ASA
http://
www.americanheart.org/presenter.jhtml?identifier=1165

The Stroke Group, Ethos II
http://www.thestrokegroup.com/

AMC Registry, Inc., The Stroke Registry
4900 Reed Road, Suite 128
Columbus, OH 43220-3164
614-457-9190 ext. 20

Stroke Sense Database
http://www.cceprograms.intranets.com

Stroke Trials Directory
http://www.strokecenter.org/

Box 2.3 Certification programs of the Association of Clinical Research Professionals

The Association of Clinical Research Professionals (ACRP) offers global certification programs as a formal recognition of clinical research professionals for clinical research coordinators (CRCs), clinical research associates (CRAs), and clinical trial investigators (CTIs). These certification examinations document the clinical research professional's knowledge and standards for professional practice. Additionally, they grant industry recognition for the clinical research professional.

To qualify for the certification examination, professionals must document a minimum of two years of full-time or four years of part-time experience enrolling subjects, conducting subject study visits, and maintaining source documents. A detailed curriculum vitae must include a description of the candidate's roles as a CRC. More information about the CCRC certification can be obtained through the ACRP website http://www.acrpnet.org/certification/fda/crc/index.html.

Benefits of CCRC certification:

- Certification is increasingly recognized by today's global clinical research industry.
- Study sites use certification for documentation to sponsors and contract research organizations (CROs) that the site is professionally managed.
- The largest investigator online databases include a request for the study coordinator's certificate number.
- Certification assists the public, health care professionals, and the industry itself by identifying standards for professional practice.

Training and professional development programs are offered through many organizations:

- The FDA (Food and Drug Administration)
- Professional membership organizations such as the Association of Clinical Research Professionals, the Drug Information Association, Regulatory Affairs Professional Society
- Private continuing education companies who sponsor conferences, offer self-study training packages, and develop training materials

Administrative assistant

Once the program grows, it is essential to budget for a position to support the activities of the stroke team.

Liaison team members

- Neuroscience unit nurse manager.
  In most centers, the stroke nurse coordinator does not function as the nurse manager for the

neuroscience unit. The stroke coordinator and the nurse manager for the unit need to work very closely to ensure clinical quality and maintenance of the expertise of the nurses staffing the stroke center.
- Rehabilitation services.
  It is productive to identify one person from the rehabilitation department to be a member of the stroke program team for the purposes of communication back to the therapists and nurses in the rehabilitation department.
- Marketing.
  Internal and external marketing are very important to the success of the stroke program. Having a dedicated person from the marketing department attached to the stroke program team is a big asset. Telling the stories of patients who have had good outcomes is a powerful marketing and educational technique. Permission to tell the story can be obtained while the patient is still in the hospital.
- Human resources (HR).
  There will be personnel issues that impact the stroke program and a liaison from HR familiar with the stroke center is key to successful resolution of these issues.
- Foundation.
  A liaison to the hospital foundation, if there is one, can be instrumental in helping raise funds for research and education projects.

In larger programs, many people from multiple departments are involved in the operations of the stroke program, and most of these people are managed through their own departments. However, there are some positions in the program that logically report to the stroke program administrator, as illustrated in the organizational chart (Figure 2.2).

MEETINGS

Planning

In the planning phase of the stroke center described in Chapter 1, the medical director, nurse coordinator, and administrator will constitute the core leadership team, and will generally meet weekly. It is important to have one meeting where everyone potentially involved in the stroke program comes together to 'dream ... what does the best possible stroke program for us look like?'. Once the scope of

Figure 2.2

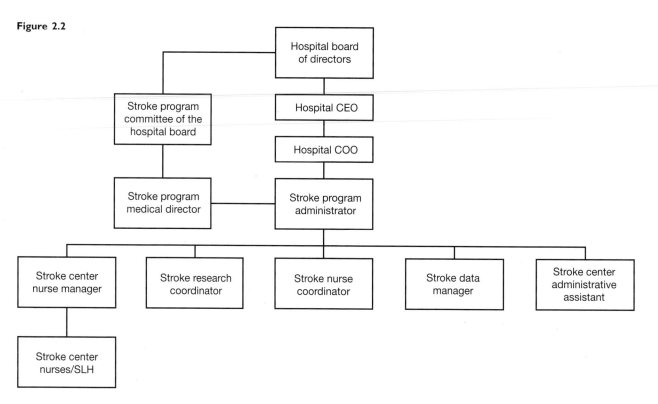

Stroke program organizational chart

the program is determined, the planning team will need to communicate with representatives from the departments involved in the care of the stroke patients. Achieving a balance between getting input from key clinicians and technicians with minimal disruption of their clinical activities is the challenge. One way to approach this is to have the core team concentrate on one department at a time. For example, when the planning involves ED operations, the core team can meet with the representatives from the ED to discuss the pertinent issues. This same process can occur with key physicians and personnel in neurology, neurosurgery, pharmacy, lab, radiology, rehabilitation services, marketing, etc.

When there are overlapping issues – e.g. stocking tissue plasminogen activator (tPA) in the ED – then representatives from pharmacy and ED can both meet with the core team. This process will protect the time of the people in the various departments. Only the core team will participate in all of the meetings. It is very important to circle back and make sure that the results of the planning are communicated back to the entire department (e.g. ED) for comments and suggestions. The core leadership team functions as the communication hub,

getting input from all the departments and clinicians and communicating back.

Clinical operations

Meetings to discuss clinical operations are generally already established in most hospitals. The neuroscience department meetings and the morbidity and mortality conferences, for example, can serve as a forum for discussion of stroke center clinical issues, difficult or interesting cases, and review of data regarding complications, outcomes, and volumes. These meetings will be attended by members of the clinical team and core leadership team (Figure 2.1) as well as the data manager. High-volume acute stroke intervention centers find it useful to review all of the interventional cases on a weekly basis.

Stroke program operations

After the program is up and running it is useful to have a monthly meeting of the key people involved in the stroke program. The core leadership team (medical director, nurse coordinator, administrator) plus the data manager, research coordinator(s) and representatives from the nursing staff of the stroke center, marketing, the hospital foundation, and rehabilitation department might constitute the stroke program operations team. Discussions regarding the clinical, research, and educational activities and reports from the data manager, marketing, and foundation representative could be regular agenda items. This team could be responsible for setting yearly goals for the stroke program and evaluating whether these are achieved. Stroke program clinicians could look to this operations team to solve problems they identify. The SWAT Team (see Appendix to this chapter), organized to identify and manage in-hospital strokes, is an example of the operations team devising a process to address an issue raised by a concerned clinician.

Board committee

If the stroke program has a committee of the board of the hospital attached to it, then meeting with that committee once or twice a year to report activities is very important.

THE PLACE

The complete spectrum of care for the stroke patient is going to occur in multiple locations in the medical center: ED, operating room, interventional radiology suite, intensive care unit, step down unit, medical/surgical hospital unit (stroke center), rehabilitation unit, and outpatient offices. The excellent outcomes for stroke patients in dedicated units do not depend on the physical space, but on the expertise of the staff and the standardized protocols for care. Nurses in all of the units need stroke education and, ideally, NIHSS certification (Appendix).

Stroke center beds

Once the patient is ready to be cared for on a medical/surgical unit, it is worthwhile to have a specified place where stroke patients go. This could be accomplished by simply designating some number of beds on a given unit as the 'stroke center beds.' Even in large-volume centers, 8–10 beds are generally enough. This way, nursing expertise can be

achieved by training a core number of stroke center nurses, and protocols and standing orders can be used routinely. The patient to nurse ratio on this unit should be no more than 4 or 5:1. If stroke patients are scattered throughout the general units of the hospital it is almost impossible to achieve the nursing expertise and routine use of standardized tools. Stroke center beds should always have cardiac monitoring available, as unsuspected arrhythmias are common in stroke victims.

Stroke center work

- Prevent complications
  - aspiration pneumonia
  - DVT and PE
  - UTI
- Determine the cause of the stroke with diagnostic studies
- Address secondary prevention
- Institute early rehabilitation.

By concentrating the patients in one location, the nurses become familiar with neurological evaluation and the diagnostic workup for stroke. This knowledge is helpful in communicating with families and referring physicians and can potentially decrease length of stay. For example, if the nurse is aware that the physician would like to order an echocardiogram if the carotid artery evaluation is unremarkable, this could be accomplished without the physician having to return to the unit. Both studies might be accomplished in one day.

It is important to have a sign identifying this part of the unit as the stroke center. A poster size version of the stroke clinical path can be hung on the wall. It helps the staff as well as the patients and their families know that something unique for the care of stroke is going on in this place.

Note: In this era of shortage of hospital beds, it must be clear that if the stroke center beds are not occupied by stroke patients, then other patients can be placed there. However, stroke patients take priority.

Step down unit

A step down unit where staffing levels would be 3:1 (patients/nurse) is a very useful concept for the care of stroke victims. Patients who have had acute stroke intervention, carotid stenting or uncomplicated clipping of an aneurysm may not need ICU level care, but need closer observation than in the stroke center, where nurses are caring for five patients. The care in the step down unit could include frequent neurological assessment, careful blood pressure monitoring, and intravenous (IV) drip therapy for blood pressure and glucose control.

THE TOOLS

The purpose of all of the tools is to standardize care as much as possible: prevent complications, institute early rehabilitation, perform appropriate diagnostic studies, identify issues in secondary prevention, assure that appropriate treatment is given, and communicate effectively with patients, families, and referring physicians.

Care paths

Stroke paths can be organized in days or phases (Appendix). Ideally, the path is initiated in the ED and carries through the ICU, stroke center and interfaces with a stroke rehabilitation care path. Usually, the path is a tool used by nurses rather than physicians and can be used as a nursing charting tool to avoid double documentation. The path can also be the source for documenting specific data elements such as verification that stroke education and information on smoking cessation were provided to the patient.

Paths for ischemic and hemorrhagic stroke may differ from paths for subarachnoid hemorrhage and TIA. Many centers develop 'patient paths' that track the same information but in lay terminology for patients and families. The paths should be reviewed annually by the stroke team nurse coordinator to be sure that they are based on current evidence.

Standing order sets

If the care paths are for nurses, the correlating tools for physicians are the standing order sets. Ideally, each path has an associated order set. The first order on stroke standing orders should be: 'Initiate stroke care path.' This automatically sets into motion the measures to prevent complications and initiate early rehabilitation. There is sometimes resistance on the part of physicians to use standing order sets. However,

no diagnostic test is done or medication given without specific orders from the attending physician. Once physicians become familiar with use of the order set, they find it saves time. It is very important when developing these orders to write a draft version and ask the physicians who will be admitting patients with strokes to make suggestions and changes. The physicians should also be given the opportunity to review the yearly updates to the order sets.

One technique to encourage the use of order sets by physicians is to require any patient who is admitted to a stroke center bed to be on the care path. Empower the stroke center nurses and the unit secretary to place the standing orders on the chart. If physicians do not want to comply, the patient can be admitted to another unit. When it becomes obvious that the standardization of care for the stroke patient ensures shorter length of stay and improved outcomes, most physicians will agree to use the tools. They must feel, however, that they have input into the content. The medical director and nurse coordinator can facilitate communication between the attending physicians and the stroke center staff.

In addition to order sets addressing various types of strokes and TIA, it is helpful to have standing orders for blood pressure management, pre and post interventional procedures such as stenting, clipping and thrombolysis, and pre and post surgical procedures.

Protocols/flowcharts

Whenever the process of care is complex, developing a protocol or flowchart can be very helpful in making sure everything is done properly and that all the providers of care are communicating accurate information. One obvious example is the administration of tPA for acute stroke. The example of an ED flowchart shown in the Appendix puts all the pertinent information onto one page. Another example is the tracking of the neurological status of the patient over time. Most stroke centers do an NIHSS on admission, at 24 hours, and at discharge. However, more frequent evaluation of the neurological status of the patient is often critical. The Neuro Frequent Assessment Tool included in the Appendix developed by the Saint Luke's Hospital stroke team was so successfully implemented in the stroke center that it is now the tool used by all units in the hospital who need to track the neurological status of the patient such as the cardiovascular ICU and cardiac catheterization labs.

Figure A2.1 Stroke Watch Action Team (SWAT)

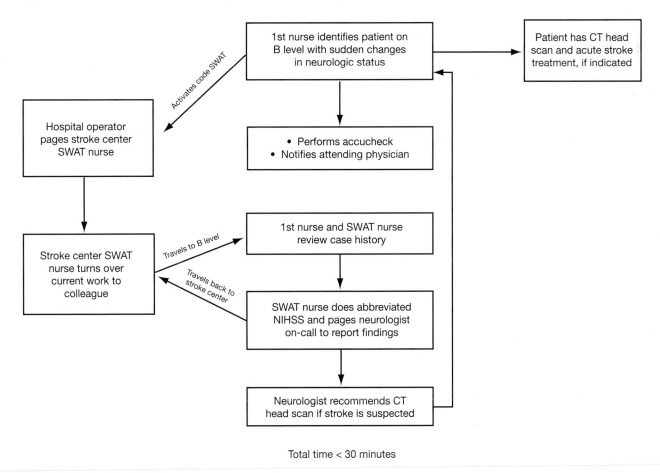

Total time < 30 minutes

Rapid identification and treatment of in-hospital strokes

Questions to consider

1. Will there be a dedicated stroke center location?
2. How many beds are required for the acute unit and step down unit?
3. Who can admit patients to the unit?
4. What policies for use of care paths and order sets will be in place on the unit?
5. What equipment is needed?
6. What will the staffing ratio be for each unit?
7. Who will train the nurses?
8. What care paths and order sets are needed?
9. Who will write the standardized tools?
10. What kind of neurological assessment will be done on the unit and how often?
11. Will all the nurses be certified to use the NIHSS?
12. Who should be on the stroke program team?
13. How often should the team meet?
14. What outcome and performance measures will be tracked?
15. What dataset will be used?

APPENDIX TO CHAPTER 2

The Stroke Watch Action Team (SWAT)

Hospitalized patients who suddenly develop symptoms of stroke need rapid assessment to determine if any intervention should be considered. The usual chain of events whereby the nurse taking care of a patient calls the house staff or attending physician can delay immediate neurological evaluation, resulting in missed opportunities for acute stroke treatment.

The Stroke Watch Action Team (SWAT) developed by the Saint Luke's Stroke Center in 1996 is a rapid response team specifically aimed at evaluating people with sudden change in neurological status. It takes advantage of the expertise of the stroke center nurses who are all trained to use the NIHSS as a tool for assessment..

Figure A2.2 (front of form)

Neurological Event				
Date: _____Time of Noted Onset: _____				
Time of Previous Assessment with No Apparent Neurological Deficits:				

PATIENT ASSESSMENT		MODIFIED NIH STROKE SCALE	* See the NIH Key on back of form	Stroke Symptoms	Recommendations
CODE SWAT TIME:				[ ] Motor	[ ] Neuro consult
BP		LOC 0-3		[ ] Sensory	[ ] CT Scan
				[ ] Language	[ ] Observation
PULSE		LOC 0-2 QUESTIONS		[ ] Visual	[ ] Heparin Drip
RHYTHM (Check one)	[ ] Irregular [ ] Regular	LOC COMMANDS 0-2		[ ] Dysarthria	[ ] ASA
				[ ] None	[ ] tPA
RESP.		MOTOR ARMS 0-4	LA	[ ] Other	[ ] Carotid Doppler
			RA	_____	[ ] Arteriogram [ ] MRI/MRA
O2 Sat		MOTOR LEGS 0-4	LL	(Check ALL that apply)	[ ] Other
			RL		[ ] None
Blood Glucose		FACIAL PALSY 0-3			(Neurologist Recommendations for Treatment)
General Patient Information		**Total**			
[ ] Recent Surgery Date:		[ ] Recent Invasive Procedure Date:			
[ ] Abdominal surgery [ ] CV Surgery [ ] Vascular surg/fem pop/ AAA		[ ] PTCA/PA [ ] Cardiac cath [ ] A-gram [ ] Other			

Reason for Admission/Diagnosis		Additional Pertinent Health History	
[ ] Arrhythmia	[ ] MI/Angina	[ ] CVA/TIA	[ ] DVT/PE
[ ] CVA/TIA	[ ] DM	[ ] CAD	[ ] CHF/Cardiomyopathy
[ ] HTN	[ ] DVT/PE	[ ] AFIB	[ ] COPD
[ ] CEA	[ ] Encephalopathy	[ ] HTN	[ ] Renal Disease
[ ] CHF	[ ] Pneumonia	[ ] DM	[ ] Abdominal Surgery
[ ] CAD	[ ] Other_____	[ ] Carotid Disease	[ ] Other_____
[ ] Renal Failure		[ ] Hyperlipidemia	

(Call 531-4080, ask office or answering service to notify on call neurologist of Code SWAT)
[ ] Dr. Arkin - 989-2203   [ ] Dr. Bettinger – 989-2198   [ ] Dr. Boutwell – 989-2205
[ ] Dr. Rymer - 989-2196   [ ] Dr. Schwartzman - 989-7819   [ ] Dr. Weinstein - 989-2197

Time Neurologist Notified:_____   Code Swat Appropriate [ ] YES [ ] NO
Comments:_____

Patient Label   Signature

RN Activating Code SWAT _____

SWAT RN _____

Original: Chart   Copy: SWAT Satchel

Patient assessment and form to be completed by SWAT RN

Code SWAT (Figure A2.1)

- Patient develops sudden change in neurological status
- Floor nurse caring for the patient needs assistance in sorting out what is going on
- Floor nurse calls hospital operator to page a code SWAT

- Floor nurse checks patient's glucose level
- One of the stroke center nurses who is working a regular shift is carrying the SWAT beeper
- Stroke center SWAT nurse turns over any work anticipated in the next 20 minutes to a colleague
- SWAT nurse picks up a bag of equipment and SWAT flowsheet (Figure A2.2) and goes to the room of the patient in question

Figure A2.2 (back of form)

FREQUENT NEUROLOGICAL ASSESSMENT KEY

LOC (Level of Consciousness)

0 = Fully alert, immediately responsive to verbal stimuli; is able to cooperate completely.

1 = Drowsy; consciousness is slightly impaired; arouses when stimulated verbally or after shaking; responds appropriately.

If the patient scores either 2 or 3 in this section of the neuro check, proceed to the Glasgow Coma Scale

2 = Stuporous; aroused with difficulty, often painful stimuli must be applied; arousal usually incomplete; responds inadequately; reverts to original state when not stimulated.

3 = Comatose; unresponsive to all stimuli or responds with reflex motor or autonomic effects.

LOC QUESTIONS

0 = Patient knows his age and the month (only initial answer is scored).

1 = Patient answers one question correctly.

2 = Patient unable to speak, to understand or answers incorrectly to both questions.

LOC COMMANDS

0 = Patient grips hand and closes/opens eyes to command.

1 = Patient does one correctly.

2 = Patient does neither correctly.

MOTOR: ARM (Right & Left)

The patient is examined with arms outstretched at 90° if sitting, or at 45° if lying down. Request full effort for 10 seconds. If consciousness or comprehension is abnormal, cue patient by actively lifting arms into position as the request for effort is verbally given.

0 = No drift (Limb holds at 90° if sitting, at 45° if lying down for full 10 seconds).

1 = Drift (Limb holds position, but drifts before 10 seconds; does not touch the bed).

2 = Some effort against gravity (Limb falls to the bed before the full 10 seconds)

3 = No effort against gravity (Limb falls, no effort against gravity, some voluntary movement observed).

4 = No movement.

U = Untestable due to amputation.

MOTOR: LEG (Right & Left)

While supine, the patient is asked to maintain the leg at 30° for five seconds. If consciousness or comprehension are abnormal, cue patient by actively lifting leg into position while the request for effort is verbally given.

0 = No drift (Leg holds 30° for five seconds).

1 = Drift (Leg falls to intermediate position by the end of five seconds).

2 = Some effort against gravity (Leg falls to bed by five seconds).

3 = No effort against gravity (Leg falls to bed immediately, with no resistance to gravity, some voluntary movement observed).

4 = No movement.

U = Untestable due to amputation.

FACIAL PALSY

Ask the patient to show teeth, raise eyebrows, squeeze and shut eyes.

0 = Normal

1 = Minor

2 = Partial

3 = Complete

- SWAT nurse discusses situation with floor nurse and gets a quick history: atrial fibrillation, glucose, recent surgery or procedure, etc.
- SWAT nurse does an abbreviated NIHSS (Figure A2.2)
- SWAT nurse pages neurologist on call with 911 after the page
- Parallel to these activities, the floor nurse has notified the attending physician/house staff of the course of events
- Neurologist answers page and discusses case with SWAT nurse
- Neurologist makes recommendation: If the case does sound like a possible stroke, the recommendation is to obtain a CT scan
- The SWAT nurse then returns to the stroke center
- The floor nurse communicates the recommendation to the attending physician who generally then orders the CT scan and, usually, a STAT neurological consultation

- The CT scan is done on a STAT basis, and the neurologist can make a recommendation as to how to treat the patient.

Since its inception in 1996, there have been 40–70 SWAT calls per year. Initially, the stroke center nurses were unsure of their skills in assessment and communication to the neurologists, but over time they have proved to be very accurate. The floor nurses are very satisfied that they now have a method to get an immediate evaluation of their patients. Concerned families are very satisfied with the quick response and evaluation for intervention. Clearly, not all the calls are actual strokes and not all of the strokes can be treated, but the process has elevated the level of care and all patients who are eligible receive treatment. Nurses, physicians, and house staff new to the hospital are educated about the services of the SWAT team.

3

Regional stroke networks

Organizing regional networks linking primary care hospitals and physicians to comprehensive stroke centers staffed and capable of providing the entire spectrum of acute stroke intervention will be essential to substantially increase the number of stroke victims who receive acute interventional therapy.

- Successful stroke intervention is time-dependent
- Stroke victims will most often go to or be taken to the closest hospital
- Hospitals will have varying capability to render acute stroke intervention.

One of the first steps in organizing a stroke center is to determine the level of care that can be provided, as discussed in Chapter 1. Once that decision is made then a logical next step is to find out the capabilities of other hospitals in the region and determine where your center fits in the spectrum of services available in these hospitals. The most likely pattern is that there will be one or more comprehensive stroke centers in the large urban center, surrounded by hospitals capable of primary stroke care, surrounded by hospitals that will be bypassed or will quickly transfer all acute stroke victims.

The most sophisticated treatments for stroke such as embolectomy, intra-arterial thrombolysis or aneurysm clipping and coiling require a neuro-interventional or neurosurgical team. This would mean that both the hospitals capable of administering intravenous (IV) thrombolytics and the hospitals without that capability should be linked to a comprehensive stroke center to provide the best possible outcome for each patient.

Some countries such as Canada and Germany have already developed regional referral networks. In the US, states including Florida, Massachusetts, New York, Texas, Maryland, New Jersey, and New Mexico are in various stages of organizing regional stroke care.

A well-established model exists in the Greater Cincinnati/Northern Kentucky region, where the acute stroke team has been available on-call 24 hours per day and 7 days per week since 1988. Emergency department (ED) physicians call the stroke pager (immediately upon patient arrival and prior to receiving CT scan and laboratory results) and speak directly to a stroke physician on-call, who immediately travels to that hospital if the patient may be an acute treatment candidate. Many patients are treated by the stroke team member at the hospital where they presented. They are followed for 24 hours by the acute stroke team, and the remainder of the hospitalization is handled by the local neurologist. However, if after acute assessment, it is determined that the patient requires the resources of a tertiary care center, the stroke physician initiates transport of the patient by helicopter or ambulance. Over 900 calls were fielded in 2004, with one-third of the cases being evaluated in person. Almost half of those seen in the EDs received acute stroke treatment.

LINKS IN THE CHAIN OF SUCCESSFUL STROKE INTERVENTION

Public awareness

Many stroke victims do not experience pain and because the brain is the affected organ they cannot process what is happening. It is usually someone else on the scene that recognizes the signs of stroke. It is important for everyone, not just the 'at risk population' to know the warning signs of stroke and to

Figure 3.1

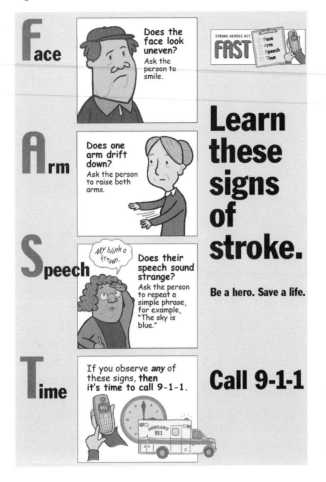

Public awareness campaign using the acronym FAST. Produced by the Heart Disease and Stroke Prevention and Control Program, Massachusetts Department of Public Health, with funding from the US Centers for Disease Control and Prevention.

know that calling 911 is the best course of action. Stroke center personnel are often the source of this education within a community. In Cincinnati, the stroke team developed a public awareness campaign using the acronym FAST to be used in evaluating a possible victim of stroke: F for face, A for arms, S for speech, and T for time (Figure 3.1).

Emergency medical services (EMS)

EMS providers play a key role in the success of acute stroke intervention. While on the scene, they can determine the time of onset and perform a quick neurological assessment such as the Cincinnati Prehospital Stroke Scale (CPSS) or the Los Angeles Prehospital Stroke Screen (LAPSS) (Appendix). They are highly accurate in making a diagnosis of stroke when using these tools. They can notify the hospital of their impending arrival so that the ED can be 'stroke ready.'

EMS are locally organized. In most communities, stroke victims are taken to the closest hospital. However, EMS crews are becoming very sophisticated regarding stroke intervention, and some will direct patients to the best hospitals for acute stroke care when asked. Rural EMS providers who are familiar with services provided by comprehensive stroke centers (CSCs) may recommend that they do not stop at the local hospital but transport by ambulance to a place where the helicopter can take the patient directly to the CSC. Some regions are formally organizing the EMS transport of stroke victims using both ambulances and helicopters.[1,2] It is important for stroke centers to become familiar with the local EMS providers. Offer education about stroke if it is needed and understand the policies that determine where stroke victims are routed in your region.

Primary hospital evaluation

The 'stroke ready' primary hospital will either be able to administer IV tissue plasminogen activator (tPA) within one hour after arrival or will have a rapid transfer protocol in place. Administering IV tPA requires that the CT scan is done and interpreted, the laboratory studies are complete, and the pharmacy is available to mix the drug. A tPA checklist is helpful to make sure that the patient is an appropriate candidate. A flowsheet can be very helpful. The example in the Appendix from the Saint Luke's Hospital Stroke Center has two possible paths. If the patient presents within 2 hours of symptom onset, then the primary hospital capable of administering IV tPA can follow that pathway. If the patient presents within 5 hours of symptom onset, there is still an option for intra-arterial interventional treatment and the transfer protocol should be instituted. These times may be lengthened again with the window of treatment for mechanical embolectomy extending to 8 hours. Some ED physicians are comfortable administering IV tPA with consultation from a neurologist. If none is available to see the patient, the consultation can be done by phone or telemedicine.[3] Many more patients could be treated within the 3 hour time window for IV tPA if there were a mechanism for quick access to a neurologist at the stroke center hospital. After administration of IV tPA the transfer protocol can still be carried out if further intervention is indicated.

There are many aspects of acute stroke care in addition to whether or not thrombolysis should be administered. These are discussed in Chapter 6 and are also very important for the primary hospital to consider.

Rapid communication and transport to comprehensive stroke center

Stroke victims who present within 5–6 hours after symptom onset may benefit from stroke intervention. The primary hospital will benefit greatly by having a relationship with a CSC. It is critical that the CSC make communication and transport very efficient. Some programs have a stroke pager that the primary hospital can access directly. The Saint Luke's system has developed a very efficient transfer team. All referring physicians/hospitals can use one phone number to transfer a patient or to speak to a stroke neurologist. The phone number accesses a trained triage nurse who asks a series of questions regarding time of onset, availability of CT scan, etc. The transfer nurse then pages the neurologist on call with a 911 page. The neurologist gets the information from the nurse and calls the referring ED to discuss options, including making a decision as to whether or not to give IV tPA in the ED at the primary hospital. If the patient is to be transferred, the stroke neurologist speaks to the patient or family by phone to discuss what might happen after transport and gets a cell phone number so that further discussion can occur after the patient arrives by ambulance or helicopter. The family always arrives later by car, and that time interval is critical. The neurologist then notifies the transfer team nurse to alert the neuro-interventional team. Everyone is ready to go once the patient arrives (Figure 3.2).

This discussion has focused on treatment for acute ischemic stroke. With new time-dependent treatments for hemorrhagic stroke such as using recombinant factor VII within 4 hours of onset, regionalization of care becomes even more important.

A CASE STUDY: THE SAINT LUKE'S HOSPITAL STROKE CENTER REGIONAL NETWORK EXPERIENCE

Since opening in 1993, the Saint Luke's Stroke Center (SLSC) has developed a relationship with many hospitals in the region. Stroke center physicians and nurses provide on-site stroke education to the staffs of these hospitals. A packet of information for the EDs has been developed (Appendix):

Figure 3.2

Regional stroke transfer

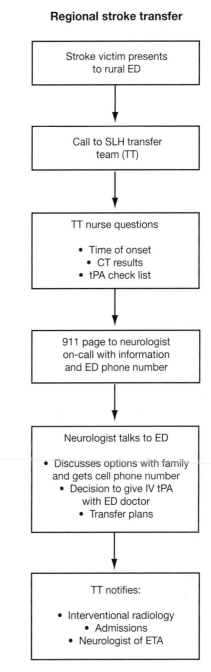

Regional stroke transfer algorithm

- Current options for acute stroke intervention
- tPA dosing charts (e.g. 0.9 mg/kg or 0.6 mg/kg)
- Rapid transfer information
- ED flowsheet.

After the patient is treated at SLSC every effort is made to get information on the outcome back to the referring ED physicians and EMS crews. This regional organization of care has resulted in a 20–30% stroke intervention rate.

Table 3.1 Ischemic stroke intervention at Saint Luke's Hospital 2004

	n	%
Ischemic strokes	514	
Stroke interventions*	144	28 (144/514)
Number of interventions that were transfer cases	101	70 (101/144)
IV tPA before transfer	50	50 (50/101)
Not transferred	43	30 (43/144)

*IV tPA, IA tPA, IV + IA tPA, mechanical embolectomy ± tPA.
(IV, intravenous; tPA, tissue plasminogen activator; IA, intra-arterial).

The results from 2004 are summarized in Table 3.1. The overall intervention rate was 28%, and 70% of those cases were referred in from 1 of 47 referring regional hospitals. Half of the referred cases received IV tPA in the local hospital before transfer, the so-called 'drip and ship' process. Mortality rates and good outcomes as indicated by NIHSS of 0–5 at discharge are similar in the patients who were transferred and those who presented primarily (no transfer) to Saint Luke's Hospital (SLH)[4] (Figure 3.3).

If it had not been for the regional network, 43 patients would have been treated rather than 144. No matter how sophisticated the level of care offered by the CSC, the patients have to arrive in time. Regional networks are critical to achieving the goal of increasing the number of stroke victims who receive treatment.

REFERENCES

1. Riopelle RJ, Howse DC, Bolton C et al. Regional access to acute ischemic stroke intervention. Stroke 2001; 32; 652–5.
2. Silliman SL, Quinn B, Huggett V, Merino JG. Use of a field-to-stroke center helicopter transport program to extend thrombolytic therapy to rural residents. Stroke 2003; 34; 729–33.
3. Wang S, Gross H, Lee SB et al. Remote evaluation of acute ischemic stroke in rural community hospitals in Georgia. Stroke 2004; 35; 1763–8.
4. Rymer MM, Thrutchley DE. Organizing regional networks to increase acute stroke intervention. Neurol Res 2005; 27(Suppl 1): S9–S16.

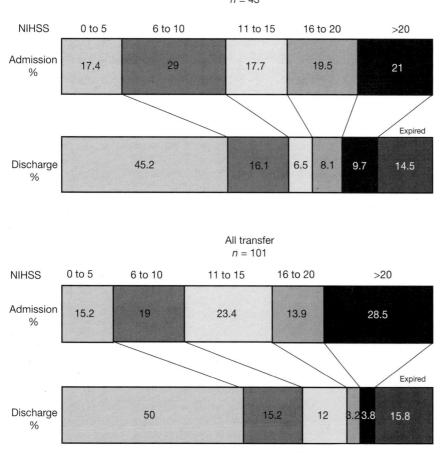

Figure 3.3 Comparison of outcomes: transfers vs not transferred

4

Imaging for diagnosis and selection of therapy

IMAGING FOR ACUTE ISCHEMIC STROKE PRESENTING WITHIN THREE HOURS

Immediate access to imaging is essential for determining if the stroke is hemorrhagic or ischemic and, thereby, planning appropriate acute therapy. The only necessary imaging modality for acute stroke treatment is the noncontrast CT (NCCT) scan. It should be available 24 hours per day and 7 days per week. The CT scan should be performed within 25 minutes of arrival and, therefore, a technician must be available promptly. In addition, interpretation must be available within 45 minutes. In many instances, the interpretation is done immediately by the physician making the decision regarding the use of thrombolytic therapy, i.e. the neurologist or emergency department (ED) physician. The need for rapid ED assessment and specific time goals are discussed further in Chapter 5.

Newer imaging modalities under development for emergent acute ischemic stroke evaluation include additional CT-based, as well as MRI studies. Advantages and disadvantages of each imaging modality will be discussed.

Emergent noncontrast CT scan

Key data provided by the NCCT scan that will influence emergent management of the stroke are:

- Ruling out intracranial hemorrhage (ICH) – the only absolute contraindication for acute ischemic stroke therapy
- Assessing for regions of clear hypodensity that would lead the clinician to reconsider the

Figure 4.1

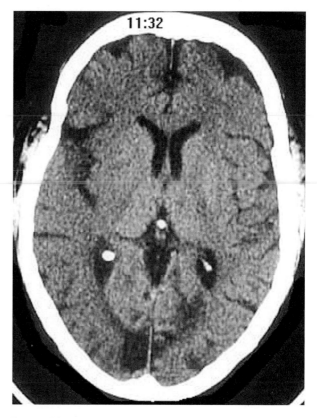

Right middle cerebral artery distribution hypodensity

accuracy of reported stroke onset timing (Figure 4.1), as well as the possibility of a recent ischemic stroke within the last 3 months (an absolute exclusion criterion).

Other findings on NCCT include the observation of a hyperdense artery (Figure 4.2), a sensitive but nonspecific sign for a large artery occlusion that may

Figure 4.2

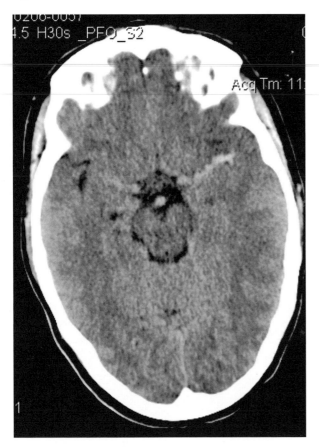

Hyperdense left middle cerebral artery (MCA)

enhanced CT sequences – the CT source images (CT-SI) from which CT angiography (CTA) is derived and CT perfusion (CTP) studies – could provide valuable information. It remains to be seen, however, whether they improve patient selection for ischemic stroke therapy and, thereby, warrant delay of treatment by approximately 30–35 minutes[2] within the 3-hour time window. At this time, obtaining this additional data is not routinely recommended for patients who can be treated within 3 hours.

CT-SI and CT perfusion studies together may offer the following:

- Quantitative maps of cerebral perfusion assessed by parameters of mean transit time (MTT), cerebral blood flow (CBF), and cerebral blood volume (CBV)
- Low CBV, specifically, may estimate irreversible ischemic injury (similar to DWI-MRI discussed below) and predict poor outcome despite recanalization[3]
- Identification of reversible ischemic tissue may be determined (based on a decreased CBF, elevated MTT, and normal or elevated CBV).

CTA may have a role in identifying subsets of patients with large artery occlusions who should receive intra-arterial (IA) therapeutic modalities in addition to, or instead of, intravenous (IV) therapy.

influence the diagnosis. Early ischemic changes, including loss of gray-white differentiation, sulcal effacement, and basal ganglia obscuration, have been quantified through a 10-point scoring system called the Alberta Stroke Programme Early CT Score (ASPECTS). In the NINDS trial, there was a trend towards reduced mortality and increased benefit to tPA (tissue plasminogen activator) with ASPECTS >7.[1] While potentially prognostically significant, these changes have not been shown to predict hemorrhagic transformation after thrombolytic therapy within three hours. Whether early ischemic changes should influence therapeutic decisions remains to be determined.

Additional CT-based imaging

CT-based technology is easily accessible, relatively rapid, and cost-effective. In addition to standard NCCT, additional CT-based imaging using contrast-

MRI modalities

Emergent MR is likely to be less accessible than CT imaging at most hospitals, but remains a promising avenue for diagnosis and therapy selection. As with CT perfusion studies, if the patient can be treated within 3 hours of symptom onset, delaying therapy by performing an MRI is not recommended.[4]

MR modalities offer the following key advantages and disadvantages:

1. Diffusion-weighted imaging (DWI)
   - High sensitivity and specificity for detecting acute ischemia[5]
   - Helpful for determining the timing of a recent stroke (i.e. whether or not the stroke occurred within the last 7–10 days) when interpreted using apparent diffusion coefficient (ADC) maps, which are derived from DWI data

- May estimate irreversible ischemia, although reversal of diffusion restriction can be achieved in some patients with effective and timely recanalization.

2. Perfusion-weighted imaging (PWI)
   - An estimate of perfusion status using MTT and CBF parameters
   - Regions of brain tissue with normal DWI and increased MTT or decreased CBF may represent regions of oligemia and reversible ischemia
   - Potential role to assess response to revascularization therapy.

3. Gradient-echo (GRE)
   - While more sensitive in detecting ICH, it remains to be seen whether hemorrhages present on GRE, but not head CT, are relevant for acute treatment decision-making. For example, studies regarding the risk of increased post-revascularization ICH in the setting of microbleeds have had mixed results.[4]

4. MR angiography (MRA)
   - As with CTA, MRA may identify subsets of patients who should receive IA therapy in addition to, or instead of, IV therapy.

IMAGING FOR ACUTE ISCHEMIC STROKE PRESENTING BEYOND THREE HOURS

Patients who cannot be treated within 3 hours of symptom onset with IV tPA may still have salvageable brain tissue. A major goal in acute stroke research is to determine a physiologic time window in which brain tissue perfusion may be critically low, but irreversible damage has not occurred.

Possible strategies to assess the degree of mismatch between irreversible ischemia and areas of critically decreased blood flow include:

- CT–clinical mismatch (i.e. the discrepancy between the apparent infarct size based on early ischemic changes on NCCT, and the extent of injury expected based on clinical examination)
- CT perfusion-based mismatch
- MR-based diffusion–perfusion mismatch.

While intuitively compelling and used as a decision-making tool in some specialized centers, the concept of preservation of mismatched oligemic, ischemic tissue remains to be proven.

IMAGING FOR SECONDARY STROKE PREVENTION

Internal carotid artery (ICA) evaluation

Assessing ICA stenosis:

- Carotid ultrasound (CUS) is an excellent screening tool. It is reasonably sensitive and specific (80–95% and 95–99% for ICA stenosis >70%; 100% sensitive and specific for occlusion), and cost-effective.[6]
- MRA 3D time of flight (TOF) has a comparable profile, but less specificity (90%) for ICA stenosis. It is dependent on flow-related signal changes and subject to velocity and turbulence alterations rather than anatomic depictions of luminal contrast. In other words, stenoses may be overestimated. However, gadolinium-enhanced MRA may improve specificity.[7] When an MRI is already being performed for other reasons, addition of MRA is a logical screening method.
- CTA is not generally used as a screening modality because it introduces the unnecessary risk of contrast toxicity and is currently less established. It is dependent on software reconstruction algorithms. However, at some centers, it is used effectively with accuracy comparable to MRA.[8]
- Digital subtraction angiography is not used for screening, due to the risk of complications in <1% of patients, unless there is another reason for performing angiography. It is primarily used when there are discrepancies between other noninvasive methods.

Identifying extracranial artery dissection:

- An MRI and MRA of the neck are warranted. A dissection protocol, consisting of T1 axial, fat-saturated MR images of the neck, should be performed. This specific sequence allows an intramural thrombus to be more easily visualized, compared with other MR sequences.

Intracranial stenosis evaluation

- CTA is reported to be highly sensitive and specific for proximal intradural intracranial stenoses. However, distal vasculature may be difficult to visualize.

- Data comparing MRA and CTA are limited. MRA, as with extracranial ICA assessment, has comparable characteristics but may overestimate stenoses. Gadolinium-enhancement may improve upon this.
- Transcranial doppler (TCD) can be used to assess only the proximal vessels in the anterior circulation and has variable accuracy in the posterior circulation, limiting its utility in this setting.[4]

REFERENCES

1. Demchuk AM, Hill MD, Barber PA et al. Importance of early ischemic computed tomography changes using ASPECTS in NINDS rtPA Stroke Study. Stroke 2005; 36(10): 2110–15.
2. Sa de Camargo EC, Koroshetz WJ. Neuroimaging of ischemia and infarction. NeuroRx 2005; 2: 265–76.
3. Wintermark M, Reichhart M, Thiran JP et al. Prognostic accuracy of cerebral blood flow measurement by perfusion computed tomography, at the time of emergency room admission, in acute stroke patients. Ann Neurol 2002; 51(4): 417–32.
4. Hjort N, Butcher K, Davis SM et al. Magnetic resonance imaging criteria for thrombolysis in acute cerebral infarct. Stroke 2005; 36: 388–97.
5. Gass A, Ay H, Szabo K, Koroshetz WJ. Diffusion-weighted MRI for the 'small stuff': the details of acute cerebral ischemia. Lancet Neurol 2004; 3: 39–45.
6. Filis KA, Arko FR, Johnson BL et al. Duplex ultrasound criteria for defining the deverity of carotid stenosis. Ann Vasc Surg 2002; 16: 413–21.
7. Pedraza S, Silva Y, Mendez J et al. Comparison of pre-perfusion and postperfusion magnetic resonance angiography in acute stroke. Stroke 2004; 35: 2105–10.
8. Koelemay MJ, Nederkroom PJ, Reitsma JB, Majoie CB. Systematic review of computed tomographic angiography for assessment of carotid artery disease. Stroke 2004; 35: 2306–12.

5

Acute stroke interventions

The availability of treatment for acute stroke, in addition to supportive care and rehabilitation, has been a major driver in the efforts to organize and standardize stroke care. Organized stroke centers will provide the critical infrastructure to implement and disseminate new therapies as they become available. This chapter discusses some of the acute treatment options that are currently being used or tested.

ISCHEMIC STROKE

The basic challenge in ischemic stroke is to restore blood flow to the brain before there is irreversible tissue damage. The most effective therapies will likely be a combination of pharmacologic and mechanical means of restoring flow while protecting brain tissue.

Intravenous tPA

Thrombolytic revascularization with intravenous (IV) tPA was the first proven, effective way to reverse neurological deficit in acute ischemic stroke.[1] For every eight people treated with IV tPA, one additional patient will have minimal or no disability. Moreover, for every three treated, one additional patient will have less disability.[2] The benefit of tPA is seen in all subtypes of ischemic strokes despite an increased risk of symptomatic intracranial hemorrhage (ICH) of 6.6%, compared with 0.6% in placebo controls, within 36 hours. This benefit of tPA administration has been reproduced by community experience.[3]

Emergency departments (EDs) are often faced with the challenge of administering IV tPA without adequate neurological support. Ideally, a hospital faced with an acute stroke treatment candidate would have a relationship with a stroke specialist by phone, video telemedicine, or in person to provide guidance (Chapter 3). Without this support, the ED physician is left with the option of developing skills to treat with tPA independently, or triaging acute stroke candidates to other hospitals, preferably before arrival to their ED so that time is not lost.

Timing: the earlier the better

Intravenous thrombolysis should be administered to all eligible ischemic stroke patients within 3 hours of stroke onset. Outcomes improve significantly with faster treatment.[4] A patient is 2.8 times more likely to achieve minimal or no disability when treated within 90 minutes of stroke onset, compared to 1.5 times more likely if treated at 91–180 minutes. Post hoc analyses suggest benefit, although diminished, beyond 3 hours from symptom onset. However, treatment beyond 3 hours is not approved therapy and should only be considered in carefully selected cases (Chapter 4).

Table 5.1 Odds ratio for favorable outcome (modified Rankin scale 0–1) at 3 months after IV tPA

Time (min)	Odds ratio (95% CI)
0–90	2.8 (1.8–4.5)
91–180	1.5 (1.1–2.1)
181–270	1.4 (1.1–1.9)
271–360	1.2 (0.9–1.5)

Rapid assessment goals

In order to increase the number of acute stroke patients receiving treatment, goals for ED assessments have been recommended as a guide. Patients should be treated with IV tPA within one hour of presentation at the emergency department (i.e. door-to-needle time).

NINDS time recommendations[5] are as follows:

1. A physician should evaluate a stroke patient within 10 minutes of arrival at the ED doors
2. A physician with expertise in the management of stroke should be available or notified within 15 minutes of patient arrival. Depending on the protocol established this may be accomplished by activating a stroke team
3. A CT scan of the head should begin within 25 minutes of arrival. The CT interpretation should be obtained within 45 minutes of arrival. Many centers are now sending patients directly to CT imaging if they are medically stable. The patient can then be brought back to the ED for the remainder of the assessment while the images are being processed
4. IV tPA treatment should be initiated within 60 minutes. But keep in mind that the earlier the treatment, the better the outcome
5. The time from patient arrival at the ED to placement in a monitored bed should not exceed 3 hours.

Pre-tPA evaluation

Good outcomes with IV tPA are dependent on following the inclusion and exclusion criteria established in the NINDS tPA trial.[1] The most important eligibility criteria are:

- Ischemic stroke causing disabling neurologic deficit
- Time of onset <3 hours. IV tPA must be administered within 3 hours of onset of symptoms. The time of onset is the last time the patient was known to be normal. A patient who went to bed at 11 pm and awakened with stroke symptoms at 6 pm is assumed to have onset 7 hours earlier and therefore is NOT eligible for tPA
- CT head scan negative for blood. This is the only absolute CT exclusion. If an area of clear hypodensity is seen, it is important to recheck the time of onset. If the hypodensity is present within 3 hours, it is generally an indication of a severe stroke. These cases carry a higher incidence of hemorrhage but hypodensity is NOT an absolute exclusion criterion
- Blood pressure ≤185/110 at the time of tPA administration without aggressive antihyperten-

sive management. Options for treatment of blood pressure include:
- Labetolol bolus of 10–20 mg over 1–2 minutes. If inadequate response within 10–20 minutes, may repeat with additional bolus, using double the prior dose
- Nitropaste 1–2 inches.

See Chapter 6 for more extensive discussion of BP management.

Additional exclusions:

- Intracranial or intraspinal surgery, serious head trauma or previous stroke within the last 3 months
- History of intracranial hemorrhage
- Major surgery within the last 14 days
- Suspicion of subarachnoid hemorrhage on pretreatment evaluation
- Arterial puncture at non-compressible site
- Active internal bleeding
- Intracranial neoplasm (except meningioma) or arteriovenous malformation (AVM)
- Known bleeding disorder: platelets <100,000; INR >1.7; elevated PTT

Relative exclusions:

- Rapidly resolving neurologic deficit. This exclusion should be carefully evaluated and has caused some confusion. Unless the rapid resolution is resulting in a very minimal deficit, treatment should still be considered
- Presumed pericarditis, including pericarditis after acute myocardial infarction
- Gastrointestinal (GI) or urinary tract hemorrhage within 21 days
- Seizure at onset
- Glucose <50 or >400
- Frank hypodensity on CT (risk of hemorrhage increases to 16%[6])
- Pregnancy.

ED evaluation:

- Confirm diagnosis and onset time; perform NIHSS
- Secure two IV lines avoiding glucose in solutions; 0.9% normal saline (NS) at 75–100 ml/h unless contraindicated
- Nasal O_2 if oxygen saturation <95%

- Brain CT
- Stroke team activation
- Electrocardiogram
- Weigh patient or estimate weight
- Accucheck
- STAT laboratory tests
  - serum electrolytes
  - glucose
  - creatinine
  - complete blood count with platelets
  - international normalized ratio (INR)
  - activated partial prothrombin time (PTT)
  - pregnancy test in selected patients
- Treat blood pressure to required level
- Discuss treatment options with family including risks and benefits. No special consent is needed for standard IV tPA therapy
- If Foley catheter is needed, insert prior to treatment.

Glucose and platelet counts should be reviewed in all patients. If there is no clinical history suggesting coagulopathy, then tPA administration should not be delayed waiting for the INR and PTT results.

This process can be greatly aided by an ischemic stroke/tPA flowsheet or checklist in the ED (Appendix).

IV tPA administration and dosing

While eligibility is being determined, tPA should be prepared. If the patient is not ultimately eligible for tPA, the cost of the tPA will be reimbursed by Genentech as per the package insert. tPA should be diluted 1:1 in sterile water or normal saline, and the mixture should be gently swirled, but not agitated. The approved dose is 0.9 mg/kg with 10% administered as a bolus over 1–2 minutes, followed by a 60 minute infusion of the remainder. Some centers are using 0.6 mg/kg with 15% administered as a bolus and the rest over 30–40 minutes if the patient is going to be considered for subsequent treatment with an intra-arterial approach. Valuable time can be saved if tPA can be kept in the ED.

Post tPA management

- Admit to an intensive care unit or a stroke unit
- Perform neurological assessments and blood pressure checks every 15 minutes for the first 2 hours, every 30 minutes for the next 6 hours, then every hour for the next 16 hours. Then every 4 hours
- If the SBP >180 or DBP >105, recheck within 5 minutes. If it remains elevated, emergently treat with antihypertensive medications (Chapter 6). 180/105 is the target BP after tPA administration
- Evaluate for angioedema q 20 minutes × 4 starting with infusion
- Provide maintenance rate of normal saline IV fluid (with NO dextrose)
- Keep the patient's head of bed flat if tolerated
- No anticoagulants or antiplatelet agents for 24 hours
- Maintain NPO until swallowing has been adequately assessed
- If the patient develops severe headache, acute hypertension, nausea, vomiting, drowsiness, or a worsening of the neurological exam, discontinue the infusion (if agent is still being administered) and obtain a CT scan of brain on an emergent basis
- Provide aggressive hyperglycemic control (Chapter 6)
- Provide mechanical deep venous thrombosis (DVT) prophylaxis
- Order a head CT for 24 ± 6 hours after the tPA was administered.

Management of complications

Angioedema:

- Incidence: estimated 1–2% of all tPA-treated stroke[7]
- Common in patients taking ACE inhibitors
- Usually starts near end of tPA infusion
- No standard guidelines available for management

Greater Cincinnati/Northern Kentucky Stroke Team Angiodema Protocol

a. Begin examining tongue 20 minutes before IV tPA infusion is completed, and repeat several times until 20 minutes after tPA infusion. Look for any signs of unilateral or bilateral tongue enlargement
b. If angioedema is suspected immediately:
   1. Consider early discontinuation of tPA infusion
   2. Benadryl 50 mg IV
   3. Ranitidine 50 mg IV or famotidine 20 mg IV
c. If tongue continues to enlarge after a–b, give Solumedrol 80–100 mg IV

d. If any further increase in angioedema:
1. Epinephrine 0.1% 0.3 ml SC or by nebulizer 0.5 ml
2. Call ENT/anesthesiology/or appropriate in-house service STAT for possible emergent cricotomy/tracheostomy or fiberoptic nasotracheal intubation if oral intubation is unsuccessful (Figure 5.1).

Figure 5.1

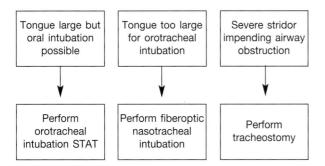

Intubation strategies in the setting of angioedema

Intracranial hemorrhage:

- Incidence: 6.6% of patients receiving IV tPA[1] Modified NINDS ICH Management Protocol
  a. Discontinue tPA infusion if still running
  b. STAT CT head scan
  c. STAT lab for type and cross, prothrombin time, PTT, platelet count and fibrinogen level
  d. Give 6 units of platelets and either 5–6 units fresh frozen plasma or 6–8 units cryoprecipitate containing factor VIII
  e. Consult neurosurgery for consideration of hematoma evacuation.

Intra-arterial tPA

Randomized evidence has shown that patients may benefit from intra-arterial (IA) thrombolytic administration, using recombinant pro-urokinase (r-pro-UK), up to 6 hours from stroke.[8] This therapy was not FDA-approved due to concerns regarding baseline group imbalances and r-pro-UK is not available commercially. Many centers are using tPA off label for IA thrombolysis. This approach may be considered in patients who arrive beyond 3 hours and can be treated by 6 hours from stroke onset. IA therapy is generally considered in patients with NIHSS ≥10 presenting after 3 hours from stroke

onset, since these patients are likely to have a visualized clot.[9,10]

Combination IV and IA tPA

Another approach for patients with moderate to severe strokes (NIHSS ≥10), administering low-dose IV tPA (0.6 mg/kg) followed by IA therapy (up to 22 mg), has been evaluated in Phase I and II trials. It is now being compared to standard IV tPA therapy in a randomized, Phase III trial.[11,12] This approach allows for early initiation of revascularization therapy while preparing for IA tPA, or device use. This lower dose of IV tPA is often the preferred approach when treatment is initiated by a referring hospital in the 'drip and ship' scenario described in Chapter 3. Some centers, however, use full-dose (0.9 mg/kg) IV tPA prior to IA therapy.

Mechanical devices

The MERCI Retriever®, a nitinol coil retrieval device evaluated in Phase I and II trials, is the first FDA-approved device for use as a method for clot

Figure 5.2

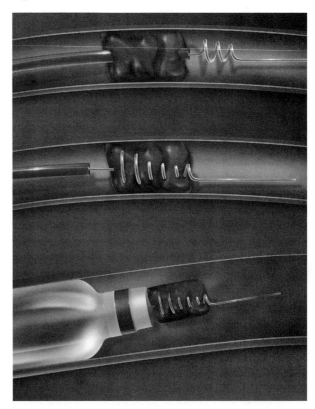

The MERCI Retriever® (Concentric Medical)

extraction in patients who are not tPA candidates or who have failed IV tPA therapy (Figure 5.2).[13] The device may be an option for anticoagulated or postoperative patients who are high risk for complications with tPA. In addition, large clots that are particularly difficult to treat with tPA might be debulked with the MERCI retriever, and followed by IA tPA to complete revascularization. Data on this approach are continuing to evolve.[14]

Another IA mechanical approach evaluated in Phase I and II trials[10] is the EKOS MicroLySUS Catheter, which can administer tPA with concurrent IA low-energy ultrasound. It has been FDA-approved for delivery of IA contrast.

Both the EKOS and MERCI devices will be further evaluated for clinical efficacy in future Phase III, randomized trials.

The use of transcranial Doppler ultrasound to enhance the lytic activity of IV tPA is also a promising avenue based on Phase II trials.[15]

Neuroprotection

Despite disappointing early trials, neuroprotection remains an area of great interest. If brain tissue could be made more resistant to injury, then there might be a longer window of opportunity for revascularization and decreased functional deficit. It is likely that there will be effective pharmacologic and mechanical neuroprotection strategies, such as the use of hypothermia.

The future

There will be new pharmacologic agents and devices for revascularization as well as effective neuroprotective strategies. These will only be successful in making an impact on stroke morbidity and mortality if the infrastructure for rapid transport and treatment is in place.

INTRACEREBRAL HEMORRHAGE

Except for removal of rapidly expanding life-threatening hematomas such as in the cerebellum, there has been no effective acute treatment for intracerebral hemorrhage (ICH). That situation is likely to change in the near future. It is well documented that ICH expands in the first 24 hours.[16] If that expansion could be limited or eliminated, the morbidity from ICH could be substantially reduced. Recombinant factor VIIa showed promising Phase II results[17] and

a larger, randomized, Phase III trial is in progress. This will also be time-dependent therapy with administration of the drug within 3–4 hours of symptom onset. Success will be dependent on the same organization of stroke care required for acute ischemic stroke treatment. Chapter 6 addresses general management of ICH.

SUBARACHNOID HEMORRHAGE

Definitive treatment of the aneurysm underlying SAH should generally be performed early.[18] Neurosurgical clipping and endovascular coiling are both options for securing a ruptured aneurysm:[19,20]

- Neurosurgical clipping
  - Preferred method of treatment until recently
  - High rate of efficacy (i.e. permanent occlusion in >90%)
  - Significant risk of morbidity and mortality (5–15%)
- Endovascular coiling
  - More recently established as an option[21]
  - More likely to result in a favorable outcome[21]
  - Possible lower rate of efficacy.[9,21]

In many cases, the two methods are complementary, with one being better than the other for an individual circumstance. Both treatments should be carefully considered by physicians with a multidisciplinary perspective.[19,22] Considerations include:

- The patient's age and medical status
- Surgical accessibility of the aneurysm
- Vascular anatomy
- Aneurysmal and parent vessel morphology
- Characteristics of the hemorrhage.

When patients are equally good candidates for either intervention, endovascular coiling is often the preferred approach.

REFERENCES

1. Tissue plasminogen activator for acute ischemic stroke. The National Institute of Neurological Disorders and Stroke rt-PA Stroke Study Group. N Engl J Med 1995; 333(24): 1581–7.
2. Saver JL. Number needed to treat estimates incorporating effects over the entire range of clinical

outcomes: novel derivation method and application to thrombolytic therapy for acute stroke. Arch Neurol 2004; 61(7): 1066–70 [Erratum in: Arch Neurol 2004; 61(10): 1599].

3. Graham GD. Tissue plasminogen activator for acute ischemic stroke in clinical practice: a meta-analysis of safety data. Stroke 2003; 34(12): 2847–50.

4. Hacke W, Donnan G, Fieschi C et al; ATLANTIS Trials Investigators; ECASS Trials Investigators; NINDS rt-PA Study Group Investigators. Association of outcome with early stroke treatment: pooled analysis of ATLANTIS, ECASS, and NINDS rt-PA stroke trials. Lancet 2004; 363(9411): 768–74.

5. Marler JR, Jones PW, Emr W. Proceedings of a National Symposium on Rapid Identification and Treatment of Acute Stroke. Bethesda, MD: The National Institute of Neurologic Disorders and Stroke (NINDS), National Institutes of Health. 1997; 97: 4239.

6. The NINDS t-PA Stroke Study Group. Intracerebral hemorrhage after intravenous t-PA therapy for ischemic stroke. Stroke 1997; 28(11): 2109–18.

7. Hill MD, Barber PA, Takahashi J et al. Anaphylactoid reactions and angioedema during alteplase treatment of acute ischemic stroke. CMAJ 2000; 162(9): 1281–4.

8. Furlan A, Higashida R, Wechsler L et al. Intra-arterial prourokinase for acute ischemic stroke. The PROACT II study: a randomized controlled trial. Prolyse in acute cerebral thromboembolism. JAMA 1999; 282(21): 2003–11.

9. Lewandowski CA, Frankel M, Tomsick TA et al. Combined intravenous and intra-arterial r-TPA versus intra-arterial therapy of acute ischemic stroke: Emergency Management of Stroke (EMS) Bridging Trial. Stroke 1999; 30(12): 2598–605.

10. Ernst R, Pancioli A, Tomsick T et al. Combined intravenous and intra-arterial recombinant tissue plasminogen activator in acute ischemic stroke. Stroke 2000; 31(11): 2552–7.

11. IMS Study Investigators. Combined intravenous and intra-arterial recanalization for acute ischemic stroke: the Interventional Management of Stroke Study. Stroke 2004; 35(4): 904–11.

12. The IMS II Investigators. Preliminary results of IMS II Trial. Stroke 2006; 37: 708.

13. Smith WS, Sung G, Starkman S et al; MERCI Trial Investigators. Safety and efficacy of mechanical embolectomy in acute ischemic stroke: results of the MERCI trial. Stroke 2005; 36(7): 1432–8.

14. Wade S, Smith CA; for the Multi-MERCI Investigators. Results of the Multi-MERCI Trial. Stroke 2006; 37: 711.

15. Alexandrov AV, Molina CA, Grotta JC et al: CLOTBUST Investigators. Ultrasound-enhanced systemic thrombolysis for acute ischemic stroke. N Engl J Med 2004; 351(21): 2170–8.

16. Brott T, Broderick J, Kothari R et al. Early hemorrhage growth in patients with intracerebral hemorrhage. Stroke 1997; 28(1): 1–5.

17. Mayer SA, Brun NC, Begtrup K et al; Recombinant Activated Factor VII Intracerebral Hemorrhage Trial Investigators. Recombinant activated factor VII for acute intracerebral hemorrhage. N Engl J Med 2005; 352(8): 777–85.

18. Whitfield PC, Kirkpatrick PJ. Timing of surgery for aneurysmal subarachnoid haemorrhage. Cochrane Database Syst Rev 2001; (2): CD001697.

19. Wijdicks EF, Kallmes DF, Manno EM et al. Subarachnoid hemorrhage: neurointensive care and aneurysm repair. Mayo Clin Proc 2005; 80(4): 550–9.

20. Suarez JI, Tarr RW, Selman WR. Aneurysmal subarachnoid hemorrhage. N Engl J Med 2006; 354(4): 387–96.

21. Molyneux A, Kerr R, Stratton I et al; International Subarachnoid Aneurysm Trial (ISAT) Collaborative Group. International Subarachnoid Aneurysm Trial (ISAT) of neurosurgical clipping versus endovascular coiling in 2143 patients with ruptured intracranial aneurysms: a randomised trial. Lancet 2002; 360(9342): 1267–74.

22. Suarez JI, Tarr RW, Selman WR. Aneurysmal subarachnoid hemorrhage. New Engl J Med 2006; 354(4): 387–96.

6

Issues in acute management

All of the following physiologic parameters are very important in the management of acute stroke. Evidence regarding optimal management will continue to evolve. A standardized approach using a care path and standing orders is the best way to make sure that all patients receive the best care. Each year, the most current evidence should be reviewed and the path and orders updated.

GLUCOSE CONTROL

Hyperglycemia predicts a worse outcome for stroke victims. The tight glucose control (80–110) that has been shown to benefit patients in the critical care literature[1] will likely translate to the stroke population, although conclusive evidence is not available. The 2003 recommendation by the American Association of Clinical Endocrinologists (AACE) calls for the upper limit of blood glucose for patients in the intensive care unit (ICU) to be 110 mg/dl. The Ischemic Stroke Pathway developed by NINDS recommends a range of 70–120 mg/dl.[2]

Hyperglycemia may be an indication of previously undiagnosed diabetes, but may also occur as a stress response. HbA1C should be checked in patients with hyperglycemia.

Management of glucose

- Normal saline instead of D5W1/2 NS should be used for intravenous (IV) fluid replacement unless there is a medical contraindication.
- If the initial glucose level is >150 mg/dl then initiate an insulin drip protocol (Box 6.1)[3] and set a target glucose range (i.e. 80–110 mg/dl or 70–120 mg/dl).

Box 6.1 Hyperglycemia treatment protocol[3]

1. Bedside blood glucose (BG) monitoring every hour until the patient is within target range on two consecutive readings, and then obtain BG every 2 hours. If the BG falls above or below the target range, resume hourly readings

2. If initial BG >150 mg/dl, give IV regular insulin bolus. Dose _____ units (dose 0.1 units/kg body weight)

3. Insulin drip: 125 units of regular insulin in 250 ml of 0.9% normal saline (1 ml of solution = 0.5 units of insulin)

4. Target BG range on insulin drip _____ mg/dl to _____ mg/dl (suggested 80–110 for ICU patients)

5. For each BG value, recalculate drip rate and disregard previous rate of infusion

6. Calculate insulin drip rate: (BG – 60) × _____ multiplier = units of insulin per hour (×2 to determine ml per hour)

7. Typical starting multiplier 0.02, but varies by insulin sensitivity
   Adjusting multiplier:
   BG > target range: increase multiplier by 0.01
   BG within target range: no change in multiplier
   BG < target range: decrease multiplier by 0.01

8. Treating hypoglycemia:
   BG 60–80: give 50% dextrose in water using formula: (100 – BG) × 0.3 = D50W IV push
   BG < 60: give D50W using formula: (100 – BG) × 0.3 = ml D50W IV
   Push and decrease insulin drip to 50% of current infusion rate
   Recheck BG in 30 minutes
   BG > 80: decrease multiplier by 0.01 and then return to step 5 formula
   BG 60–80: Repeat step 8 with BG 60–80
   BG < 60: notify physician and repeat step 8 with BG < 60

9. Special considerations:
   Tube feeding adjustments: notify physician to determine adjustments of insulin for interruption of feedings for traveling to or having procedures

---

Note: There are devices in development that can be implanted subcutaneously for real-time continuous glucose monitoring. There are no data available yet regarding their use in stroke victims.

TEMPERATURE CONTROL

Hyperthermia also predicts worse outcomes for stroke victims. It has not yet been determined if hypothermia is beneficial, but there are some data to indicate that this might be the case.

Management of temperature

- Normothermia should be maintained using acetaminophen. In the acute setting, delivery by mouth may not be desirable, so rectal suppository or nasogastric tube are the preferred routes of administration. This can be a standing order in the acute stroke order set.
- If normothermia cannot be maintained with acetaminophen, a cooling blanket may be used.
- If hyperthermia continues, a source of infection should be evaluated and treated appropriately.
- Numerous systems that induce hypothermia are in development and testing.[4]

OXYGEN SATURATION

Oxygen saturation should be maintained >95% with the administration of O_2 via nasal cannula.

CARDIAC TELEMETRY

Cardiac telemetry is indicated for all stroke victims for 24–72 hours to detect arrhythmias. In patients with atrial fibrillation, the telemetry can be used to ensure adequate heart rate control.

HEAD OF THE BED

Ideally, patients with ischemic stroke and a perfusion deficit should have the head of bed FLAT for at least 12 hours. Airway patency and risk of aspiration have to be factored into this decision. After 12 hours, the head of the bed can be raised to 30°. Frequent neurological assessment should be done after raising the head of the bed. If any deterioration is noted, the bed should be lowered to a flat position for at least 6 hours. In patients with hemorrhagic stroke, the head of the bed should be at 30° if there are any clinical or radiographic signs of increased intracranial pressure.[5]

BLOOD PRESSURE CONTROL

Blood pressure (BP) management is, perhaps, the most important of all the parameters. Target BP will be different depending on the type of stroke, and evidence will continue to evolve. This is an area where the stroke team needs to review the literature regularly so that targets can be revised based on new information. The goal is to maintain maximum cerebral perfusion while minimizing the risk of hemorrhage or extension of hemorrhage. In complicated cases where there is hypertensive encephalopathy, acute myocardial infarction (MI), aortic dissection, acute renal failure or hemorrhagic transformation of ischemic stroke, target BPs will have to be lower than the following recommendations.

- Ischemic stroke treated with thrombolysis. BP must be <185/110 prior to treatment with tissue plasminogen activator (tPA) and be maintained at <180/105 for 24 hours post tPA therapy. This translates to a mean arterial pressure

> **Box 6.2 Options for management of hypertension**
>
> - Labetolol 10–40 mg bolus over 1–2 minutes. Repeat for two or three doses to target BP. Total dose should not exceed 100 mg in one period of treatment and should not exceed 300 mg per day. Cautions: asthma, chronic obstructive pulmonary disease (COPD), left ventricular (LV) failure, second or third degree heart block, heart rate <50.
> - Nicardipine drip 5 mg/h IV infusion. Increase by 2.5 mg/h every 5 minutes to a maximum of 15 mg/h to achieve target BP. Cautions: LV failure, aortic stenosis, cardiac ischemia.
> - Nitroprusside 0.25–10 µg/kg/min. This is not recommended unless control cannot be achieved with other agents or the level of hypertension is extreme. Cautions: elevated ICP, coronary artery disease, renal insufficiency.
> - Hydralazine 10–20 mg IV every 4–6 hours. Cautions: ischemic heart disease, aortic dissection, mitral valve disease.
> - Enalaprilat 0.625–1.2 mg IV every 6 hours. Cautions: acute MI, history of angioedema, renal insufficiency.

of 130 (2 × diastolic + systolic divided by 3). Protocols and agents for managing hypertension are summarized in Box 6.2. It is just as important to treat low BP to maintain perfusion pressure. When clinical instability appears to be due to hypotension, a target mean arterial pressure (MAP) of 120–130 can be achieved with fluid boluses and titrating a neosynephrine drip at 0.5–3 μg/kg/ min. This should be used with caution in patients with congestive heart failure, coronary artery disease or renal insufficiency.

- Ischemic stroke not treated with thrombolysis.
  In the first 24 hours after acute stroke, hypertension should not be treated unless SBP >220, DBP 121–140 or MAP >130 on two consecutive readings at least 5 minutes apart. Treatment should be initiated with labetolol 10–20 mg IV over 1–2 minutes or nicardipine 5 mg/h infusion as initial dose, titrated to the target BP by increasing 2.5 mg/h every 15 minutes to a maximum of 15 mg/h. Patients with SBP >220 and DBP >140 should receive sodium nitroprusside 0.25–10 μg/kg/min via arterial line even though it may aggravate or produce increased intracranial pressure (ICP).[6] In most cases, BP will spontaneously decrease over the first 24 hours and a gradual decrease of 15% is desirable. BP can then be gradually lowered to a normal range when the perfusion deficit has cleared. This can be assessed with a perfusion scan or assumed to be the case in 5 days.

- Intracerebral hemorrhage.
  American Stroke Association Guidelines recommend that BP be maintained below a MAP of 130 (180/105). If an ICP monitor is in place, BP should be titrated to maintain cerebral perfusion pressure >70 mmHg.[7] If surgical evacuation occurs, MAP of > 110 should be avoided in the immediate postoperative period. If systolic pressure falls to <90, neosynephrine or dopamine drip should be instituted. The goal is to minimize hematoma enlargement. Some centers set a target MAP of <120.

- Subarachnoid hemorrhage (SAH).
  BP management after SAH is complex because of the need to balance the risk of rebleeding with the need to maintain perfusion pressure in infarcted brain. In all cases, avoid SBP <100 for 21 days. Before repair of the aneurysm, SBP should be ≤160. Should symptomatic vasospasm occur, some evidence would support increasing

SBP to a maximum of 200–220.[8] The specific target BP and optimal agents for treatment after SAH vary between centers and clinicians. Some experts advocate not treating until MAP is >130, while others aggressively maintain SBP at <140 to 160 mmHg.

ANTITHROMBOTICS IN ACUTE ISCHEMIC STROKE

Despite their frequent use, there is no evidence that antithrombotics are beneficial in the treatment of acute ischemic stroke. This holds true even for subcategories such as suspected cardioembolic stroke, progressive hemispheric stroke, basilar thrombosis, and carotid or vertebral artery dissections. Despite the lack of evidence there are some situations in which the use of anticoagulants might be considered in the acute setting in patients with minor (small) infarctions:

- High risk for deep vein thrombosis (DVT)
- Identified potential cardiac source of embolus
  - Atrial fibrillation
  - Mechanical heart valve
  - Akinetic segment
  - Mural thrombus
  - Ejection fraction <25%
  - Mitral stenosis
  - Anterior wall MI within 2 weeks
- Extracranial carotid or vertebral dissection
- Intracranial venous thrombosis
- Symptomatic high-grade carotid stenosis awaiting emergency surgery.

The potential benefits would need to be weighed against the possible risk of secondary hemorrhage. In part, this risk depends on the size of the ischemic infarction.[9]

Antithrombotics for secondary stroke prevention are discussed in Chapter 8.

INTRACRANIAL PRESSURE

Patients with small to moderate-sized strokes usually do not have significantly increased ICP. However, multilobar hemispheric infarction and large brainstem or cerebellar infarctions or hemorrhages are at risk for increased ICP and/or hydrocephalus. Increased ICP carries a risk of cerebral herniation.

ICP pressure generally peaks at 72 hours after a stroke.[10]

Signs of increased ICP are:

- Change in level of consciousness (LOC)
- Agitation
- Pupillary changes such as unilateral dilation
- Change in respiratory pattern
- Increased BP
- Decreased pulse rate
- Decerebrate posturing.

In hemorrhagic stroke, an ICP monitor should be placed in patients with a Glasgow Coma Scale (GCS) <9 or in patients who are clinically deteriorating. A ventricular drain should be placed if hydrocephalus is present. The target ICP is <20 mmHg for all patients.

If ICP is increased, hypo-osmolar IV fluids such as D5W should be avoided. Other treatment modalities include:[3]

- Head of bed raised 30–45° to promote venous drainage.
- Treat fever with acetaminophen or cooling blankets to reduce metabolic demand.
- Treat agitation or cough with one of the following:
  - Propofol 1 mg/kg followed by 1–3 mg/kg/h
  - Morphine 1–2 mg IV as needed
  - Fentanyl: loading dose 50–150 μg; maintenance 30–100 μg/h.
- Mannitol 20% 0.25–0.5 g/kg every 4 hours. Serum osmolality should be measured every 6 hours and dose adjusted with target osmolality of ≤310 mOsm/L. Mannitol should be discontinued if serum sodium is >148. Treatment should not exceed 5 days and therapy should be weaned gradually to avoid rebound.
- Hyperventilate to pCO_2 of 35–30 mmHg by increasing respiratory rate to 18–20. Hyperventilation should not be maintained for more than 6 hours. Taper gradually to normal pCO_2 over 24 hours.
- Neuromuscular paralysis with sedation in patients with high ICP or those who are 'bucking' the ventilator. Vecuronium 0.02 mg/kg loading dose with infusion rate of 1 μg/kg/min.
- Moderate hypothermia (32–33°C) using cooling blankets or ice packs.
- Barbiturate coma: pentobarbital is the most frequently used agent.

In large hemispheric or cerebellar hemorrhagic strokes, emergent neurosurgical consultation should be obtained for possible decompression. In large hemispheric ischemic strokes at risk for herniation, hemicraniectomy can be considered.

Herniation can occur very rapidly. It is important to discuss treatment options with the family before the emergent situation arises. In light of a devastating stroke, sometimes the family declines intubation and invasive treatment based on the known wishes of the patient. This decision needs to be made ahead of time.

SPECIFIC ISSUES IN SUBARACHNOID HEMORRHAGE

Complications after rupture:

- Cardiac abnormalities: dysrhythmias, T wave inversion, prolonged QT interval, ST elevation
- Rebleeding (highest risk in the first 7–10 days). Early intervention with clipping or coiling may prevent rebleeding. If intervention is delayed, aminocaproic acid is used to prevent clot dissolution
- Hydrocephalus occurs in 20% of patients within 24 hours and may require ventriculostomy
- Seizures
- Vasospasm leading to infarction can occur 3–14 days after rupture. Volume expansion with triple H therapy (hypervolemia, hemodilution, and hypertension), albumin or plasma protein fraction increases cerebral perfusion. Nimodipine (calcium channel blocker) at 60 mg every 4 hours by mouth or by nasogastric tube is used to prevent vasospasm. Nimodipine should be continued for 3 weeks. Other more aggressive therapies include angioplasty and the use of papaverine. The diameter of the vasospastic blood vessel is increased with papaverine but the effect lasts less than 24 hours and there may be a toxic effect on the brain distal to the site of infusion. Angioplasty has a longer treatment effect, but vessel rupture is a potential complication. Verapamil can be injected into smaller vessels affected by vasospasm.

TRANSIENT ISCHEMIC ATTACKS

The definition of a transient ischemic attack (TIA) is in evolution. While the established definition is a transient neurological deficit lasting less than 24 hours, common experience is that most TIAs are very short. In addition, diffusion-weighted magnetic resonance (MR) images are often positive in people with TIAs. The border between TIA and mild stroke continues to blur. Both should be treated as an opportunity to prevent a larger stroke from occurring. The diagnostic evaluation of a TIA is the same as for stroke. How emergent should the evaluation be?

- 25–30% of strokes are preceded by TIAs
- After a TIA, there is a 10% chance of stroke in the next 90 days
- One-half of the strokes that occur in 90 days occur in the first 2 days following the event.

Clinical markers indicating higher risk

- Age > 60 years
- Diabetes
- TIA lasting longer than 10 minutes
- Weakness persisting after other symptoms have resolved.

Evaluation for the cause of the TIA should be accomplished expeditiously, given that the highest risk of stroke is in the first hours to weeks after the event. Carotid artery imaging to rule out high-grade stenosis should be a priority. Patients with recent symptoms of TIA or minor stroke should be hospitalized for rapid investigation of the cause. At the Saint Luke's Hospital Stroke Center, the average length of stay for TIA is 1.8 days.

REFERENCES

1. van den Berghe G, Wouters P, Weekers F et al. Intensive insulin therapy in the critically ill patients. N Engl J Med 2001; 345(19): 1359–67.
2. NIH Stroke Team Ischemic Pathway. NINDS, Bethesda, MD. August 24, 2004.
3. Paolino AS, Garner KM. Effects of hyperglycemia on neurologic outcome in stroke patients. J Neurosci Nurs 2005; 37(3): 130–5.
4. Kriger DW, De Georgia MA, Abou-Chebl A et al. Cooling for acute ischemic brain damage (cool aid): an open pilot study of induced hypothermia in acute ischemic stroke. Stroke 2001; 32(8): 1847–54.
5. Wojner-Alexander AW, Garami Z, Chernyshev OY, Alexandrov AV. Heads down: flat positioning improves blood flow velocity in acute ischemic stroke. Neurology 2005; 64(8): 1354–7.
6. Adams HP Jr, Adams RJ, Brott T et al.; Stroke Council of the American Stroke Association. Guidelines for the early management of patients with ischemic stroke: a scientific statement from the Stroke Council of the American Stroke Association. Stroke 2003; 34(4): 1056–83.
7. Schellinger PD, Fiebach JB, Hoffmann K et al. Stroke MRI in intracerebral hemorrhage: is there a perihemorrhagic penumbra? Stroke 2003; 34(7): 1674–9.
8. Rose JC, Mayer SA. Optimizing blood pressure in neurological emergencies. Neurocritical Care 2004; 1(3): 294.
9. Berge E, Sandercock P. Anticoagulant and antiplatelet treatment of acute ischemic stroke. In: Adams H, ed. Handbook of Cerebrovascular Diseases, 2nd edn. New York, NY: Marcel Dekker, 2005, pp. 390–1.
10. Krieger DW, Demchuk AM, Kasner SE, Jauss M, Hantson L. Early clinical and radiological predictors of fatal brain swelling in ischemic stroke. Stroke 1999; 30(2): 287–92.

7

Prevention of complications

Stroke centers provide organized, standardized care that results in better outcomes even when no acute therapy is rendered. Decreasing the occurrence of secondary complications through the use of clinical pathways and order sets is a major factor contributing to the improved outcomes.

There are several complications associated with stroke. These include increased intracerebral pressure with the risk of herniation (Chapter 6), aspiration pneumonia, pulmonary embolism, deep venous thrombosis (DVT), urinary tract infection, malnutrition, bowel and bladder dysfunction, joint abnormalities, seizures, and decubitus ulcers.[1] A geographically designated area to care for stroke patients with trained health care providers ensures coordinated delivery of care and enhances communication among the team of caregivers. This is the optimal setting in which to prevent secondary complications.[2,3]

SEIZURES

Seizures are reported to occur after stroke in 4–43% of cases, and are more often associated with large cortical or lobar strokes.[4] Seizures may occur at onset or develop as soon as 24 hours after stroke and 20–80% of these patients have recurrent seizures. The most common type is a simple partial seizure with or without generalization. Stroke patients should only be given anticonvulsants if a seizure occurs. There is no indication for prophylactic therapy. Patients and families should be educated that seizures may occur after a stroke.

INFECTIONS

Pneumonia and urinary tract infections are frequent complications of stroke and are a common cause of increased hospital stays and delayed rehabilitation. Infection should be suspected if the patient develops fever or a change in the level of consciousness (LOC).

Pneumonia

The most common cause of death in the first 48 hours following acute stroke is pneumonia, often related to aspiration. Pneumonia accounts for 15–25% of stroke mortalities.

Increased incidence of pneumonia occurs with:[1]

- Dysphagia – higher incidence with facial palsy and decreased LOC
- Immobility and the development of atelectasis
- Mechanical ventilation
- Brainstem strokes
- More than one infarcted territory.

Care strategies to decrease development of pneumonia:

- Nothing by mouth (NPO) until formal swallowing evaluation to assess risk of aspiration. If a speech therapist is not available, a bedside swallowing test can be done by giving the patient 3 oz of water and observing for cough, dysphonia lasting 1 minute, respiratory difficulty, or drooling. If the swallowing test is failed, place an enteral feeding tube

- Monitor airway and oxygenation and use mechanical ventilation if indicated. Hypoxia may be due to concurrent medical conditions such as hypoventilation, atelectasis, aspiration, pneumonia, or pulmonary embolism
- Minimize time on mechanical ventilation; frequent suctioning
- Early mobilization
- Good pulmonary toilet
- Position in semi-recumbent position when feeding with a nasogastric tube or percutaneous endoscopic gastrostomy (PEG) tube
- Consult a speech pathologist and dietician to establish feeding plan and safety measures to decrease aspiration risk
- Education of patient and family regarding the risk of aspiration and the importance of following the established feeding plan and safety measures (Box 7.1).

Urinary tract infection

Urinary tract infection (UTI) develops in approximately 16% of stroke patients. Indwelling bladder catheters may be necessary in the acute phase to accurately monitor output. Catheters are also commonly placed in patients with decreased LOC or severe immobility. Changes in sphincter control and the use of indwelling catheters increase the risk of UTI. Catheters should be removed as soon as the patient is medically and neurologically stable to prevent iatrogenic infection. Intermittent catheterization or acidification of the urine may lessen the risk of UTI. Urinalysis cultures should be obtained to detect UTI in the presence of fever or change in LOC and proper antibiotic treatment should be initiated.[5]

Indwelling catheters should not be used as the treatment for incontinence that occurs in 30–60% of patients during the early period of recovery.[6] A bladder program should be implemented to retrain the bladder. Preventing the bladder from filling beyond 500 ml will stimulate normal physiological filling and bladder empting. A bladder scanner must be used to assess post-void residuals (PVR) and determine the need for intermittent catheterization. Two or more PVRs of >150 ml have been found to be an independent risk factor for UTI. Urinary incontinence is associated with poor prognosis, interferes with rehabilitation, and is the major factor in patients being discharged to nursing homes rather than to their home.

Box 7.1 Dysphagia detection and aspiration prevention

Pre-printed admission order sets that include 'swallow assessment before any oral intake' and provide further direction for those patients demonstrating a dysphagia risk.

- Maintain NPO status. No ice chips; no oral medications; no water; and no exceptions!
- Speech language pathologist (SLP) evaluation formally with appropriate diagnostic tool
- Follow (SLP) recommended compensatory techniques such as:
  - Chin tuck maneuver
  - Head and neck positioning
  - Change the consistency of food – thickened liquids, pureed, semi-solid foods
  - Minimize distractions in environment when feeding
  - No use of straws
  - High Fowler's position, leave sitting up for 30 minutes
  - Place food on the unaffected side (instruct patient/care provider)
  - Present small portions; provide time to chew and swallow
  - Evaluate for pocketing of food
  - Initiate mouth care to facilitate swallowing

CONSTIPATION

Constipation is a common problem following acute stroke and is most often forgotten by the health care team (Box 7.2).[7,8]

NUTRITIONAL COMPROMISE

Malnutrition has been proven to interfere with recovery after a stroke.[9] A swallow assessment should be done as soon as possible after admission to the hospital and no later than 48 hours after admission. Nutrition should be established within 48–72 hours. Feeding through a nasogastric tube may be used initially but if dysphagia is expected to continue beyond 6–8 weeks, early gastrostomy should be considered.[10] If no dysphagia or aspiration risk is detected, oral feeding should be instituted immediately. Dysphagia resolves completely in 87% of all stroke patients. Feeding should begin as soon as possible after the patient has been cleared for risk of aspiration. Serum albumin is a poor indicator of immediate nutritional state since it has a half-life of 18 days. The dietician should be consulted early for an evaluation of nutritional status and need. Malnutrition should be prevented as it impairs the

Box 7.2 Bladder and bowel training

The program should include:
1. Bladder scanning and intermittent catheterization every 4–6 hours; continue intermittent catheterization as long as post-void residual (PVR) is > 100
2. Initiate voiding strategies
   a. Offering a commode, bedpan, or urinal every 2 hours during waking hours and every 4 hours at night. Neurological deficits lead to frequent falls when patients try to ambulate to the bathroom
   b. Assist patients with toileting when impaired vision, mobility, and dexterity are present
3. Communication boards to aphasic patients to provide quick request
4. Monitor fluid intake during the evening prior to bed
5. Evaluate for abdominal distension
6. Evaluate for impaction every 2 days
7. Integrate stool softeners, laxative, and enemas to prevent constipation
8. Skin care to decrease incidence of skin breakdown, dermatitis, or perineal thrush
9. Address psychosocial problems and decreased self-esteem associated with bowel and bladder dysfunction

immune system and increases weakness, length of stay, and mortality.[11]

DEEP VEIN THROMBOSIS AND PULMONARY EMBOLISM

Early mobility can decrease the incidence of pulmonary embolism (PE), atelactasis, pneumonia, and deep vein thrombosis (DVT). Patients should be mobilized as soon as they are hemodynamically stable. During the first 30 days, 51% of deaths are related to complications associated with immobility. The most common complication of immobility is DVT. Stroke patients with a paretic or paralyzed lower extremity have the highest risk of DVT. DVT prevalence in stroke patients ranges from 20 to 50%. Death related to pulmonary embolus occurs in 10% of stroke patients.

DVT risk stratification can be used to guide treatment (Table 7.1). Early mobilization is the most effective preventative strategy. Other strategies include:[12]

1. Thromboembolic stockings (TEDs)
2. Pneumatic compression devices
3. Unfractionated heparin 5000 units twice daily subcutaneously
4. Enoxaparin (Lovenox) 40–80 mg subcutaneously once daily.

MUSCULOSKELETAL COMPLICATIONS

The rehabilitation team should be consulted on admission to instruct the care team in how to perform passive and active range of motion and positioning techniques that can prevent joint contractures and atrophy.[13] Subluxation of the affected shoulder is very common and may not be preventable. However, careful positioning and movement of the affected arm may prevent the development of a painful shoulder-hand syndrome.

Table 7.1 Deep venous thrombosis prevention through stratification

Category	Definition	Recommendation
Low risk	Ambulatory within 24 hours of admission No lower extremity motor deficits	Encourage ambulation
Moderate risk	Non-ambulatory within 24 hours for any reason Mild lower extremity motor deficits	Venodynes (SCDs) and heparin 5000 u SQ BID
High risk	Patients with co-morbid conditions: Morbid obesity (BMI > 30) CHF (NYHA III and IV) Prior DVT or PE Postpartum Postoperative (within 1 week) Cancer (active, solid organ) Antiphospholipid antibody syndrome History of cerebral venous thrombosis	Venodynes (SCDs) and heparin 5000 u SQ TID Or IVC filter placement

BMI, body mass index; CHF, congestive heart failure; DVT, deep vein thrombosis; IVC, inferior vena cava; PE, pulmonary embolism; SCD, sequential compression device; SQ, subcutaneous.

Special care should be taken to avoid pulling on the affected arm and shoulder when repositioning the patient in bed or when assisting with transfers.[14]

FALLS

Falls are the most frequent cause of injury in stroke patients. Nurses must monitor the initial transfer from bed to upright position and checking lying and sitting blood pressure can give valuable information that will decrease the risk of falling on transfers. The most common injury is hip fracture. Hip fractures in the first 7 days post stroke are associated with a poor prognosis.[15] Most fractures occur at the time of the fall and are on the paretic side.[16] Neglect, which is typically seen with right hemispheric infarcts, leads to a higher risk of falling.

Stroke team nurses must implement a fall prevention program that includes:

- Identification of high-risk patients
- Alarm systems
- Adaptive equipment such as wedge seat cushions or enclosure beds
- Call buttons and patient's belongings should be close to the patient
- Scheduled voiding times; many falls occur as the patient is trying to go to the bathroom
- A sitter in the patient's room may be required to provide the necessary safety.[15]

All of the health care providers and the family should be made aware of the fall prevention plan.

SKIN BREAKDOWN

Stroke patients are at risk for skin breakdown because of the loss of sensation and impaired circulation. Patients at risk for pressure ulcers are usually older, have a decreased LOC, and are unable to move themselves in bed due to paralysis. Other related complications such as incontinence can accelerate the development of skin breakdown. Pressure areas include heels, sacrum, and lateral malleoli.

Strategies to prevent skin breakdown:

- Patients should be examined for pressure points and massaged when turned
- Patients should not be left in a position for longer than 2 hours

- Patient's skin must be kept clean and dry
- Special mattresses should be used to prevent the development of decubiti
- Special care should be taken when repositioning, turning, or transferring patients to avoid excessive friction or excessive pressure that may lead to skin injury.[14]

DISCHARGE PLANNING

The goal of discharge planning is to ensure safe transition from the acute setting to an appropriate setting where the patient can obtain optimal rehabilitation and further secondary stroke prevention. Continuing attention to the prevention of the complications discussed above is essential to assuring the best possible outcome. For patients with continued immobility, it is very important to continue DVT, UTI, pneumonia, and skin breakdown prophylaxis and to continue a fall prevention program. Communication of the plan implemented in the acute care setting should be provided to the extended care facility at the time of discharge.

According to the National Institute of Neurological Disorders and Stroke, 35% of stroke survivors will recover fully or only have minor impairments. However, 40% will require special care and a skilled nursing facility will be necessary for 10%. A team involving the physicians, stroke team nurse, rehabilitation therapists, case manager, and social worker must begin looking at discharge needs immediately on admission. The average length of stay of 5.3 days, according to National Center of Health Statistics, does not provide the patient or family with sufficient time to understand the impact of the stroke. The discharge team must actively involve the family and assist them in making discharge decisions based on the patient's needs and family support systems. Discharge teams should strive to obtain optimal clinical outcomes by planning for rehabilitation and prevention of recurrent stroke and complications, while being attentive to containing the financial burden for the family.

REFERENCES

1. Adams HP Jr, del Zoppo GJ, von Krummer R. Management of stroke: a practical guide for the prevention, evaluation and treatment of acute stroke, 2nd edn. Caddo, OK: Professional Communication Inc; 2002 p. 140.

2. Schwamm LH, Pancioli A, Acker JR 3rd et al.; American Stroke Association's Task Force on the Development of Stroke Systems. Recommendations for the establishment of stroke systems of care: recommendations from the American Stroke Association's Task Force on the Development of Stroke Systems. Stroke 2005; 36(3): 690–703.

3. Evans A, Perez I, Harraf F et al. Can differences in management processes explain different outcomes between stroke unit and stroke-team care? Lancet 2001; 358(9293): 1586–92.

4. Johnston KC, Li JY, Lyden PD et al. Medical and neurological complications of ischemic stroke: experience from the RANTTAS trial. RANTTAS Investigators. Stroke 1998; 29(2): 447–53.

5. Adams HP Jr, Adams RJ, Brott T et al.; Stroke Council of the American Stroke Association. Guidelines for the early management of patients with ischemic stroke: a scientific statement from the Stroke Council of the American Stroke Association. Stroke 2003; 34(4); 1056–83.

6. Gelber DA, Good DC, Laven LJ, Verhulst SJ. Causes of urinary incontinence after acute hemispheric stroke. Stroke 1993; 24(3): 378–82.

7. Chan H. Bladder management in acute care of stroke patients: a quality improvement project. J Neurosci Nurs 1997; 29(3): 187–90.

8. Patel M, Coshall C, Rudd AG, Wolfe CD. Natural history and effects on 2-year outcomes of urinary incontinence after stroke. Stroke 2001; 32(1): 122–7.

9. Daniels SK, Brailey K, Foundas AL. Lingual discoordination and dysphagia following acute stroke: analyses of lesion localization. Dysphagia 1999; 14(2): 85–92.

10. Runions S, Rodrique N, White C. Practice on an acute stroke unit after implementation of a decision-making algorithm for dietary management of dysphagia. J Neurosci Nurs 2004; 36(4): 200–7.

11. FOOD Trial Collaboration. Poor nutritional status on admission predicts poor outcomes after stroke: observational data from the FOOD trial. Stroke 2003; 34(6): 1450–6.

12. Geerts WH, Pineo GF, Heit JA et al. Prevention of venous thromboembolism: The Seventh ACCP Conference of Antithrombotic and Thrombolytic Therapy. Chest 2004; 126: 338S–400S.

13. Bernhardt J, Dewey H, Thrift A, Donnan G. Inactive and alone: physical activity within the first 14 days of acute stroke unit care. Stroke 2004; 35(4): 1005–9.

14. Brandstater ME, Shutter LA. Rehabilitation interventions during acute care of stroke patients. Top Stroke Rehabil 2002; 9(2): 48–56.

15. Kelly-Hayes M. Stroke outcome measures. J Cardiovasc Nurs 2004; 19(5): 301–7.

16. Poole KE, Reeve J, Warburton EA. Falls, fractures, and osteoporosis after stroke: time to think about protection? Stroke 2002; 33(5): 1432–6.

8

Secondary prevention of stroke

ISCHEMIC STROKE

After providing indicated acute interventions and management, the next goal of hospitalization is to determine the cause of the stroke to prevent a recurrent event.

The risk of a recurrent ischemic event is substantial. Recurrent ischemic strokes occur in 5–18% of patients (depending on the definitions used) within 90 days of the first event.[1] Transient ischemic attacks (TIAs) provide a 'warning,' the unique opportunity for intervention before a stroke occurs. Strokes occur in 10% of TIA patients within 90 days, half of whom experience the recurrent event within 2 days of the TIA.[2] Therefore, it is imperative that a diagnostic workup be initiated during the hospitalization to identify treatable causes, and that appropriate secondary prevention strategies be offered promptly.

Causes of ischemic stroke can be classified as:[3,4]

- Cardioembolism (about 20%)
- Large vessel atherosclerosis (about 15%)
- Small vessel ischemic disease (about 15%)
- Other (including iatrogenic, sickle cell disease, hypercoagulable disorders, and extracranial artery dissection) (about 5%)
- Cryptogenic (45%).

An essential stroke workup consists of the following:

- Evaluation for cardiac source of embolus
  - Echocardiography with bubble study to determine a cardiac source of direct or paradoxical embolism
    - If there is no history of heart disease, a transesophageal echocardiogram (TEE) may be the preferred test

- Telemetry to detect unsuspected arrhythmias such as paroxysmal atrial fibrillation
- Carotid artery evaluation
  - Carotid ultrasound (CUS) or neck magnetic resonance angiography (MRA) for anterior circulation strokes to rule out hemodynamically significant carotid stenosis
- Imaging of intracranial and vertebral artery anatomy with MRA or angiography to discover focal stenoses IF:
  - no carotid or cardiac cause is identified, and
  - the patient is having recurrent ischemic events in the same vascular territory
- Fasting lipids and glucose levels to diagnose hyperlipidemia and diabetes mellitus.

Other workup that may impact secondary prevention strategies in the appropriate clinical settings includes:

- T1 fat-saturated axial neck magnetic resonance imaging (MRI) sequences or conventional angiography to rule out extracranial arterial dissection
- Hypercoagulable studies to assess for coagulopathy.

Diagnostic considerations and management strategies for each of the common stroke etiologies are discussed further below.

Large artery atherosclerosis

Internal carotid artery disease

Almost all stroke patients with anterior circulation strokes should be screened for symptomatic internal carotid artery (ICA) stenosis during the hospitalization.

Without treatment, patients with >70% ICA stenosis carry a 26% risk of recurrent ipsilateral stroke over 2 years.[5]

Diagnosis
- Initial screening by CUS or MRA (Chapter 4)
- If an intervention is being considered based on screening, a second confirmatory test should always be performed to confirm the degree of stenosis
- If screening and confirmatory test results are conflicting, a digital subtraction angiogram is indicated to resolve the discrepancy.

Management
Key considerations:[6]

- If a 70–99% symptomatic ICA stenosis is identified, carotid endarterectomy (CEA) is the established therapy
  - The patient should have at least a 5-year life expectancy and the estimated risk of perioperative stroke or death should be <6%. For every six patients treated with CEA, one ipsilateral stroke will be prevented over the next 2 years. Specifically, 26% of patients without CEA vs 9% with CEA have recurrent ipsilateral strokes over 2 years (P <0.001)
- CEA may be considered for patients with 50–69% symptomatic ICA stenosis based on clinical and angiographic variables
  - Considerations include gender (women have not been shown to benefit from CEA in this circumstance), the clinical event (those with preceding hemispheric stroke or TIA are more likely to benefit), and contralateral ICA occlusion (a situation with greater perioperative risk but more persistent long-term benefit)
- CEA within 2 weeks of TIA or nondisabling stroke achieved greater benefit than waiting > 2 weeks based on post hoc data analyses, suggesting that early treatment should be offered in these clinical settings
- Aspirin therapy (81 or 325 mg) should be given prior to CEA and indefinitely thereafter
  - Data are not available regarding other antiplatelet agents in this setting.

Other considerations:

- Patients at high risk for CEA may be offered carotid stenting and should be referred to a neurointerventionalist[7]

- High-risk candidates include those with severe cardiac and pulmonary disease, age >80 years, recurrent stenosis, contralateral ICA occlusion, and prior neck surgery or irradiation, and contralateral laryngeal nerve palsy
- Whether carotid stenting is appropriate as a first-line therapy for all patients is yet to be determined. While data are pending, some believe that a nonsurgical approach to carotid artery stenosis will play a prominent role for many patients in the future
- In certain circumstances, such as a substantial infarction of the given ICA territory or poor medical or neurological status, treatment of carotid stenosis may not be warranted.

Intracranial artery stenosis

Diagnosis
- Since evidence regarding optimal management of these patients is evolving, a head MRA to screen for intracranial stenoses may define etiology but not yet direct therapy.

Management
- Aggressive risk factor management, including antiplatelet therapy, statins, and antihypertensives, is the standard of care for treatment of symptomatic intracranial stenosis
  - A randomized clinical trial has shown no benefit of anticoagulation, compared to high-dose aspirin therapy, for intracranial stenosis.[8] Therefore, long-term anticoagulation is not indicated in most circumstances
- Situations leading to consideration of less established modes of care may include:
  - Suspicion of a hemodynamically dependent lesion
  - Recurrent strokes despite maximal medical therapy referable to an intracranial stenosis
  - A suspected localization where recurrent stroke can be devastating such as a basilar artery stenosis
- Investigational modes of care include:
  - Stenting or angioplasty for intracranial stenosis
  - Extracranial/intracranial bypass in selected patients, possibly using computed tomography (CT) perfusion as a guide to which patients might benefit.

Extracranial vertebral artery stenosis

Similar considerations regarding diagnosis and management are made for vertebral artery stenosis as for intracranial stenoses. Interventional treatments are only considered in the setting of recurrent symptoms despite maximal medical therapy.

Cardioembolism

Diagnosis

- All stroke patients should be screened for a possible cardioembolic etiology if this would lead to a change in management
  - Cardioembolism should be considered regardless of the presumed stroke subtype, including strokes with a lacunar appearance on imaging, since up to 25% of presumed small vessel strokes are due to other etiologies[9]
- If a patient is already in atrial fibrillation but not optimally treated, then effective long-term anticoagulation is indicated and an echocardiogram may not be needed
- Every patient with minimal or no risk factors should be screened for paradoxical embolus with TEE and bubble study.

A cardioembolic stroke workup consists of:

- A transthoracic and/or transesophageal echocardiogram with bubble study
- Continuous telemetry monitoring for 48–72 hours for paroxysmal or undiagnosed arrhythmias.

The decision to use a transthoracic echocardiogram (TTE) versus transesophageal echocardiogram (TEE) is controversial. TEE has been suggested as a cost-effective first-line diagnostic strategy by several groups.[10,11] Others suggest that these studies did not account for increased length of hospital stay, the need for sedation, and patient discomfort that come with TEE use. A common practice is to go straight to TEE when the patient is young or without known cardiac disease and/or suspicion of a cardioembolic source is high (i.e. strokes in multiple vascular distributions, or branch distal artery infarcts without intracranial/extracranial stenoses). In others, a TTE may be done first, followed by a TEE if there are cardiac abnormalities or suspicion of cardioembolism becomes high after receiving other study results.

Common cardiac diseases associated with stroke risk are:[12,13]

- Atrial fibrillation
- Cardiac heart failure with low ejection fraction

- Patent foramen ovale with atrial septal aneurysm
- Aortic arch atherosclerosis.

Uncommon conditions include:

- A left atrial or ventricular thrombus
- Prosthetic valves
- Infective endocarditis
- Marantic endocarditis
- Intracardiac tumors.

Management

Atrial fibrillation

Anticoagulation is indicated in most patients.

- There is a 12% risk of recurrent stroke. Stroke recurrence rates are reduced to approximately 10% annually with aspirin therapy alone, compared to 4% using anticoagulation[14]
- Anticoagulation initiation in patients with acute ischemic stroke is typically delayed by a few days to 2 weeks, using clinical judgment
  - The risk of hemorrhagic conversion, based on the size of the infarct, must be balanced with consideration of potential benefit. Data are not available to guide this decision.

Congestive heart failure

Congestive heart failure (CHF) is the second most common cardioembolic etiology of stroke.

- Optimizing cardiac status through coronary reperfusion, if indicated, and pharmacological therapy should be pursued
- While controversial, anticoagulation may be considered in the setting of a suspected cardioembolic stroke with concurrent CHF.[15,16]

Patent foramen ovale with atrial septal aneurysm

Patent foramen ovale (PFO) with an atrial septal aneurysm (ASA) is associated with increased stroke risk in aspirin-treated patients less than 55 years old.

- There is currently no evidence regarding optimal treatment (i.e. use of antiplatelet therapy versus anticoagulation versus surgical or endovascular closure)[17]
- Trials investigating mechanical closure are underway
- PFO alone has not been shown to increase the risk of recurrent stroke among aspirin-treated cryptogenic stroke patients.

Severe ascending aortic arch atheroma

Severe ascending aortic arch atheroma ($\geq$4 mm, ulcerated, or mobile) is also a cardiac risk factor.[13] Optimal management of this condition (i.e. antiplatelets versus short-term anticoagulants) is unknown.

Uncommon conditions

Uncommon conditions may warrant specific treatments such as anticoagulation (left cardiac thrombus, prosthetic valves, and marantic endocarditis), intensive antibiotic therapy (infective endocarditis), and resection (intracardiac tumors).

Other causes of ischemic stroke

Less common causes of stroke, listed in order of prevalence, are:[18]

- Iatrogenic (i.e. post-surgical)
- Angiography/percutaneous transluminal coronary angioplasty (PTCA)-related
- Hypercoagulable states (including sickle cell disease)
- Extracranial artery dissection
- Cocaine or narcotic use
- Hypotension
- Cancer
- Venous sinus thrombosis
- Temporal arteritis.

Small-vessel ischemic disease and cryptogenic strokes

After the diagnostic workup, over one-half of patients have no specific etiology identified.[19] If the patient has significant vascular risk factors and a small infarct consistent with a lacune (i.e., <2 cm), the etiology is often presumed to be small vessel ischemic disease. When this is not the case, the stroke is classified as 'cryptogenic.' In either case, as with all stroke etiologies, modifiable vascular risk factors should be addressed.

Modifiable cardiovascular risk factors

Aggressive treatment of modifiable risk factors is essential for almost all stroke subtypes. Risk factors with evidence-based treatment recommendations are discussed below.[16]

Hypertension

Hypertension is the most important modifiable risk factor for stroke. Management of hypertension in the acute setting must be distinguished from long-term management goals.

Acute setting

During the acute stroke phase, mean arterial pressures (MAPs) may directly impact perfusion to ischemic and oligemic brain tissue due to loss of autoregulation of the cerebral vasculature. Blood pressure is often liberalized, although randomized clinical trial data are lacking. Specifically:

- If tissue plasminogen activator (tPA) therapy was administered, maintaining blood pressure below 180/105 for the first 24 hours after treatment is critical (Chapter 5)
- Among patients for whom an acute intervention was not used, evidence-based data are not available. Blood pressure should be allowed to run relatively high. Treating MAPs >140 may be considered[20] (Chapter 6)
- Preadmission antihypertensive agents are often held or reduced, unless they are being used for other indications such as cardiac rate control
- Limited data suggest that autoregulation remains abnormal for the next 1–2 weeks and, therefore, aggressive hypertension management may be delayed during this time.[21]

Chronic setting
- All stroke and TIA patients should be prescribed antihypertensive therapy if blood pressures are >120/80.[22] Randomized, controlled trials have shown that reduction of systolic blood pressure by >10 mmHg decreases stroke risk by 30% over about 5 years[23]
- ACE inhibitors and thiazide diuretics are recommended as first-line agents for cerebrovascular disease. ACE inhibitors or angiotensin receptor blockers (ARBs) should be used first in diabetics, due to their renal protective effects.[22]

Diabetes

Diabetes mellitus is an independent risk factor for stroke.

- All stroke patients should be screened for diabetes with a fasting glucose and Hgb A1C

- Patients with a fasting (i.e. >8 hours without PO intake) glucose ≥126 or a random plasma glucose >200 are considered diabetic, and 100–125 are prediabetic[24]
- Management of diabetes mellitus includes diet, exercise, oral hypoglycemic agents, and insulin
  - The goal is to maintain hemoglobin A1C levels ≤ 7[25]
- Whether prediabetic stroke patients should be treated with oral hypoglycemics as a secondary stroke prevention measure is currently under investigation.

Hyperlipidemia

Elevated serum triglycerides, total cholesterol, and low-density lipoprotein (LDL) are risk factors for cardiovascular disease. Their role in stroke is less established, which may reflect varying degrees of risk based on specific ischemic stroke subtypes.

- Fasting lipids should be obtained on admission or within 24 hours of admission to guide discharge medication regimens
  - Based on data from patients hospitalized for acute coronary syndromes, LDL levels drop after the first few hours following an acute event and may remain low for weeks before eventually reaching admission levels again. Therefore, repeat measurements as an outpatient should be considered[26]
- Symptomatic carotid artery disease is considered a coronary heart disease (CHD) equivalent. Atherosclerotic stroke subtypes may be considered CHD equivalents as well[16]
- Based on the presence of a CHD equivalent, the following lipid goals should be achieved:[26]
  - LDL <100
  - Non-HDL (i.e. total cholesterol minus HDL) <130
  - Triglycerides <200
- The treatment approach should start with achieving the LDL goal[26]
  - A therapeutic lifestyle change (TLC), including diet (consisting of saturated fat <7% of calories, cholesterol <200 mg/day, and 10–25 g/day of increased fiber or 2 g/day of plant stanol/sterol intake), weight management, and increased physical activity, may be considered for 3 months prior to drug therapy if the LDL is 100–129

- Initiation of drugs immediately upon diagnosis is also a reasonable approach
- Statins should be first-line drugs for stroke patients. In fact, data suggest that stroke patients may benefit from statin therapy regardless of cholesterol levels.[27]

Tobacco use

- Patients who are currently tobacco users should be strongly encouraged to quit smoking
- Even a reduction in smoking is helpful
- Limiting second-hand smoke exposure is also recommended
  - Exposure to tobacco has been shown to increase the rate of atherosclerosis accumulation[28]
- Counseling should be provided to all stroke patients who use tobacco. Support groups should be offered if available. Successful tobacco cessation requires repeated interventions
- Pharmacotherapies should be offered to all patients who are attempting to quit smoking[29]
  - First-line therapies are sustained-release bupropion hydrochloride (i.e. Wellbutrin) and nicotine products (gum, inhaler, nasal spray or patch)
  - Second-line therapies are clonidine, hydrochloride, and nortryptiline hydrochloride.

Alcoholism

Heavy drinking or chronic alcoholism is a significant risk factor, and alcohol use should be stopped or reduced to no more than two drinks per day for men and one drink per day for women.[16]

Obesity

Obesity, defined as a body mass index (BMI) >30 kg/m^2, is an independent risk factor for stroke. Weight management through balanced calorie intake, exercise, and behavioral counseling should be encouraged in all stroke and TIA patients. A goal BMI of 18.5–24.9 kg/m^2 is recommended. [16]

Exercise

Thirty minutes of moderate intensity exercise on most days is recommended for secondary stroke prevention.[16]

Antiplatelet therapy for secondary stroke prevention

Aspirin is well-established for secondary stroke prevention.

- Therapy should be started within 48 hours of stroke, and is typically started on the day of presentation, after determining that there is no ICH on the head CT
  - Early aspirin treatment leads to an absolute risk reduction in stroke recurrence of 1% in the first 2 weeks after stroke[30]
  - In the long term, among stroke and TIA patients, aspirin reduces the rate of recurrent stroke by 22% annually, regardless of dosing, from 50 to 325 mg daily doses[31]
- If the patient receives an acute reperfusion intervention, aspirin should be held until 24-hour CT results showing no hemorrhage have been obtained
- Whether the lowest effective dose is 50 versus 75 mg is debatable.[31]

Alternative agents to be considered include clopidogrel (Plavix) and an ASA/extended release (ER)-dipyrimadole combination (Aggrenox).

- Clopidogrel has been shown to reduce stroke recurrence rates comparably to aspirin
  - However, clopidogrel decreased the risk of the combined end point of myocardial infarction (MI), stroke, and vascular death by an additional 8.7% compared with aspirin, primarily due to an increased benefit in peripheral vascular disease patients[32]
  - Of note, combination therapy using both aspirin and clopidogrel offers no benefit over clopidogrel or aspirin alone, but provides added risk of life-threatening and major bleeding events[33,34]
  - Whether there may be a role for this combination immediately after an acute stroke, analogous to acute coronary stent placement, has not been investigated.
- The ASA/ER-dipyrimadole combination has been shown to lead to a 23% relative risk reduction in stroke recurrence rates, compared with aspirin[35]
  - An ongoing large trial, randomizing patients to clopidogrel versus aspirin/ER-dipyridamole therapy, is likely to be informative.

The decision regarding which antiplatelet agent to initiate after a first stroke must be individualized.

Aspirin, ER-dipyridamole, and clopidogrel are all acceptable options.[16]

- A logical approach is to prescribe the aspirin/ER-dipyridamole combination for maximal prevention after a first stroke rather than waiting for an episode of 'aspirin failure.' This strategy is likely to be cost-effective as well[36]
- Clopidogrel may be a good option for patients with known concurrent peripheral vascular disease
- Finally, for patients with concurrent cardiac disease who may require more than 50 mg of aspirin daily or for whom cost is a concern, aspirin therapy alone may be most appropriate.

Discharge instructions after ischemic stroke

In-depth education regarding secondary prevention is difficult in the acute care setting. However, at discharge, it is ideal to give the patient and family a written summary of the individual risk factors, the target for improving each risk factor, and the strategy for doing so. This should also be communicated to the primary care physician who will usually resume care of the patient.

INTRACEREBRAL HEMORRHAGE

- Uncontrolled hypertension is, by far, the most common risk factor for intracerebral hemorrhage (ICH). As in the case of ischemic stroke, the management of hypertension is usually handled differently in the acute versus chronic settings
  - In the acute setting, blood pressure management is liberalized. While evidence regarding specific parameters is lacking, guidelines suggest treating MAPs >130[37]
  - After 7–10 days, additional antihypertensives may be added or restarted
  - Strict hypertension management should be attempted within 4–6 weeks
- Amyloid angiopathy, trauma, vascular malformations, or an underlying tumor are other considerations, depending on the location and appearance of the ICH. The workup is dictated by the clinical scenario
  - Considerations include the imaging appearance of the ICH and the patient's history. For example, lobar hemorrhages warrant gradient echo (GRE) MRI imaging to look for

evidence of prior microhemorrhages. Diagnosis of amyloid angiopathy may impact the decision to use anticoagulation therapy, although definitive evidence on this topic is not available[38]

- A heterogeneous or atypical appearance of the ICH warrants an MRI to look for vascular malformations during the hospitalization. If unrevealing, another MRI should be performed after 1–2 months to reassess the appearance after blood resorption

- Clinical factors adding to suspicion of a vascular malformation, such as an MRI appearance of blood vessel feeders, a lobar location of ICH, younger age, and no history of hypertension, should raise the suspicion for an underlying vascular malformation and lead to further screening by MRA and/or cerebral angiogram.

REFERENCES

1. Coull AJ, Rothwell PM. Underestimation of the early risk of recurrent stroke: evidence of the need for a standard definition. Stroke 2004; 35(8): 1925–9.

2. Johnston SC, Gress DR, Browner WS, Sidney S. Short-term prognosis after emergency department diagnosis of TIA. JAMA 2000; 284(22): 2901–6.

3. Adams HP Jr, Bendixen BH, Kappelle LJ et al. Classification of subtype of acute ischemic stroke. Definitions for use in a multicenter clinical trial. TOAST. Trial of Org 10172 in Acute Stroke Treatment. Stroke 1993; 24(1): 35–41.

4. Flaherty ML, Kleindorfer D, Alwell K et al. Did more testing lead to fewer cryptogenic strokes during the 1990s? Stroke 2006; 37(2): 649.

5. Barnett HJ, Taylor DW, Eliasziw M et al. Benefit of carotid endarterectomy in patients with symptomatic moderate or severe stenosis. North American Symptomatic Carotid Endarterectomy Trial Collaborators. N Engl J Med 1998; 339(20): 1415–25.

6. Chaturvedi S, Bruno A, Feasby T et al.; Therapeutics and Technology Assessment Subcommittee of the American Academy of Neurology. Carotid endarterectomy – an evidence-based review: report of the Therapeutics and Technology Assessment Subcommittee of the American Academy of Neurology. Neurology 2005; 65(6): 794–801.

7. Yadav JS, Wholey MH, Kuntz RE et al.; Stenting and Angioplasty with Protection in Patients at High Risk for Endarterectomy Investigators. Protected carotid-artery stenting versus endarterectomy in high-risk patients. N Engl J Med 2004; 351(15): 1493–501.

8. Chimowitz MI, Lynn MJ, Howlett-Smith H et al.; Warfarin-Aspirin Symptomatic Intracranial Disease Trial Investigators. Comparison of warfarin and aspirin for symptomatic intracranial arterial stenosis. N Engl J Med 2005; 352(13): 1305–16.

9. Gan R, Sacco RL, Kargman DE, Roberts JK, Boden-Albala B, Gu Q. Testing the validity of the lacunar hypothesis: the Northern Manhattan Stroke Study experience. Neurology 1997; 48(5): 1204–11.

10. McNamara RL, Lima JA, Whelton PK, Powe NR. Echocardiographic identification of cardiovascular sources of emboli to guide clinical management of stroke: a cost-effectiveness analysis. Ann Intern Med 1997; 127(9): 775–87.

11. Kapral MK, Silver FL. Preventive health care, 1999 update: 2. Echocardiography for the detection of a cardiac source of embolus in patients with stroke. Canadian Task Force on Preventive Health Care. CMAJ 1999; 161(8): 989–96.

12. Kasner S, Gorelick PB, eds. Prevention and Treatment of Ischemic Stroke. Philadelphia, PA: Butterworth-Heinemann, 2004.

13. Macleod MR, Amarenco P, Davis SM, Donnan GA. Atheroma of the aortic arch: an important and poorly recognised factor in the aetiology of stroke. Lancet Neurol 2004; 3(7): 408–14.

14. EAFT (European Atrial Fibrillation Trial) Study Group. Secondary prevention in non-rheumatic atrial fibrillation after transient ischaemic attack or minor stroke. Lancet 1993; 342(8882): 1255–62.

15. Hunt SA; American College of Cardiology; American Heart Association Task Force on Practice Guidelines (Writing Committee to Update the 2001 Guidelines for the Evaluation and Management of Heart Failure). ACC/AHA 2005 guideline update for the diagnosis and management of chronic heart failure in the adult: a report of the American College of Cardiology/American Heart Association Task Force on Practice Guidelines (Writing Committee to Update the 2001 Guidelines for the Evaluation and Management of Heart Failure). J Am Coll Cardiol 2005; 46(6): e1–82.

16. Sacco RL, Adams R, Albers G et al.; American Stroke Association Council on Stroke; Council on Cardiovascular Radiology and Intervention; American Academy of Neurology. Guidelines for prevention of stroke in patients with ischemic stroke or transient ischemic attack: a statement for healthcare professionals from the American Heart Association/

American Stroke Association Council on Stroke: co-sponsored by the Council on Cardiovascular Radiology and Intervention: the American Academy of Neurology affirms the value of this guideline. Stroke 2006; 37(2): 577–617.

17. Messe SR, Silverman IE, Kizer JR et al.; Quality Standards Subcommittee of the American Academy of Neurology. Practice parameter: recurrent stroke with patent foramen ovale and atrial septal aneurysm: report of the Quality Standards Subcommittee of the American Academy of Neurology. Neurology 2004; 62(7): 1042–50.

18. Khatri P, Kissela B, Alwell K, et al. Other causes of ischemic stroke and TIA are predominantly iatrogenic. Neurology 2005; 64(Suppl 1): A402.

19. Schneider AT, Kissela B, Woo D et al. Ischemic stroke subtypes: a population-based study of incidence rates among blacks and whites. Stroke 2004; 35(7): 1552–6.

20. Adams HP Jr, Adams RJ, Brott T et al.; Stroke Council of the American Stroke Association. Guidelines for the early management of patients with ischemic stroke: a scientific statement from the Stroke Council of the American Stroke Association. Stroke 2003; 34(4): 1056–83.

21. Dawson SL, Panerai RB, Potter JF. Serial changes in static and dynamic cerebral autoregulation after acute ischaemic stroke. Cerebrovasc Dis 2003; 16(1): 69–75.

22. Chobanian AV, Bakris GL, Black HR et al.; National Heart, Lung, and Blood Institute Joint National Committee on Prevention, Detection, Evaluation, and Treatment of High Blood Pressure; National High Blood Pressure Education Program Coordinating Committee. The Seventh Report of the Joint National Committee on Prevention, Detection, Evaluation, and Treatment of High Blood Pressure: the JNC 7 report. JAMA 2003; 289(19): 2560–72 [Erratum in: JAMA 2003; 290(2): 197].

23. Lawes CM, Bennett DA, Feigin VL, Rodgers A. Blood pressure and stroke: an overview of published reviews. Stroke 2004; 35(3): 776–85 [Corrected and republished in: Stroke 2004; 35(4): 1024].

24. American Diabetes Association. Diagnosis and classification of diabetes mellitus. Diabetes Care 2006; 29(Suppl 1):S43–S48.

25. American Diabetes Association. Standards of medical care in diabetes. Diabetes Care 2006; 29(Suppl 1): S4–42.

26. Expert Panel on Detection, Evaluation, and Treatment of High Blood Cholesterol in Adults. Executive Summary of The Third Report of The National Cholesterol Education Program (NCEP) Expert Panel on Detection, Evaluation, And Treatment of High Blood Cholesterol In Adults (Adult Treatment Panel III). JAMA 2001; 285(19): 2486–97.

27. Collins R, Armitage J, Parish S, Sleight P, Peto R; Heart Protection Study Collaborative Group. Effects of cholesterol-lowering with simvastatin on stroke and other major vascular events in 20536 people with cerebrovascular disease or other high-risk conditions. Lancet 2004; 363(9411): 757–67.

28. Howard G, Wagenknecht LE, Burke GL et al. Cigarette smoking and progression of atherosclerosis: The Atherosclerosis Risk in Communities (ARIC) Study. JAMA 1998; 279(2): 119–24.

29. The Tobacco Use and Dependence Clinical Practice Guideline Panel, Staff, and Consortium Representatives. A clinical practice guideline for treating tobacco use and dependence: a US Public Health Service report. JAMA 2000; 283(24): 3244–54.

30. CAST (Chinese Acute Stroke Trial) Collaborative Group. CAST: randomised placebo-controlled trial of early aspirin use in 20,000 patients with acute ischaemic stroke. Lancet 1997; 349(9066): 1641–9.

31. Antithrombotic Trialists' Collaboration. Collaborative meta-analysis of randomised trials of antiplatelet therapy for prevention of death, myocardial infarction, and stroke in high risk patients. BMJ 2002; 324(7329): 71–86 [Erratum in: BMJ 2002; 324(7330): 141].

32. CAPRIE Steering Committee. A randomised, blinded, trial of clopidogrel versus aspirin in patients at risk of ischaemic events (CAPRIE). Lancet 1996; 348(9038): 1329–39.

33. Diener HC, Bogousslavsky J, Brass LM et al.; MATCH investigators. Aspirin and clopidogrel compared with clopidogrel alone after recent ischaemic stroke or transient ischaemic attack in high-risk patients (MATCH): randomised, double-blind, placebo-controlled trial. Lancet 2004; 364(9431): 331–7.

34. Bhatt DL, Fox KA, Hacke W et al. Clopidogrel and aspirin versus aspirin alone for prevention of athereothrombotic events. N Engl J Med 2006; 354(16): 1706–17.

35. Diener HC, Cunha L, Forbes C, Sivenius J, Smets P, Lowenthal A. European Stroke Prevention Study. 2. Dipyridamole and acetylsalicylic acid in the secondary prevention of stroke. J Neurol Sci 1996; 143(1–2): 1–13.

36. Jones L, Griffin S, Palmer S et al. Clinical effectiveness and cost-effectiveness of clopidogrel and modified-release dipyradimole in the secondary

prevention of occlusive vascular events: a systematic review and economic evaluation. Health Technol Assess 2004; 8(38): iii–iv, 1–196.

37. Broderick JP, Adams HP Jr, Barsan W et al. Guidelines for the management of spontaneous intracerebral hemorrhage: a statement for healthcare professionals from a special writing group of the Stroke Council, American Heart Association. Stroke 1999; 30(4): 905–15.

38. Towfighi A, Greenberg SM, Rosand J. Treatment and prevention of primary intracerebral hemorrhage. Semin Neurol 2005; 25(4): 445–52.

9

Stroke rehabilitation

Stroke remains the leading cause of adult disability, despite new approaches to treatment and management. Indeed, 40% of stroke patients are left with moderate functional impairments, and 15–30% with severe disability.[1] Every stroke center needs access to a multidisciplinary rehabilitation team to maximize recovery for each patient. Ideally, patients should be evaluated by the rehabilitation team as soon as they are medically stable.

The five major goals of stroke rehabilitation are as follows:[2]

1. Prevention, recognition, management, and minimizing the impact of pre-existing medical conditions.
2. Training for maximal functional independence.
3. Facilitating optimal psychosocial adaptation and coping by both the patient and family.
4. Promoting community reintegration, resumption of prior life roles, and return to home, family, recreational, and vocational activities.
5. Enhancing quality of life.

Because of the myriad of functional domains encompassed by these goals, rehabilitation relies heavily on a 'team approach,' ideally including the physiatrist, speech therapist, physical therapist, occupational therapist, neuropsychologist, social worker, recreation therapist, and others working with the patient to set goals and reintegrate the patient back into the desired community. A physiatrist is, perhaps, the most key player, as the phsyiatrist is the team leader who organizes the various components of a rehabilitation plan for a particular patient. Ironically, regular, yearly contact with the physiatrist is also often the most ignored component of a comprehensive rehabilitation plan.

While physical rehabilitation (e.g. physical and occupational therapy, spasticity management) is perhaps the most recognized facet of stroke rehabilitation, other aspects of the rehabilitative process, such as management of depression and cognitive impairments, are equally important. These deficits continue long after the usual rehabilitation process has been completed, and may involve professionals such as neuropsychologists. Participation in a stroke support group by both the patient and the caregiver can also be helpful in connecting to community resources.

In this chapter, we review the typical stroke motor recovery patterns, rehabilitation strategies for specific impairments, and some new stroke rehabilitation techniques.

The American Stroke Association Practice Guideline for the Management of Adult Stroke Rehabilitation Care is one resource that also summarizes evidence-based 'best practices' for stroke rehabilitation.[1]

ACUTE INPATIENT REHABILITATION

During acute stroke rehabilitation, the patient is ideally involved in physical rehabilitation as soon as medical stabilization occurs. Acute rehabilitation is also ideally directed at preventing secondary complications, including the occurrence of another stroke. All of these aspects of care should be included in the clinical pathway. Programs in acute rehabilitation should not only include physical, occupational, and speech therapy, but should also evaluate:

- Medical problems
- Mental status
- Sensation
- Skin integrity
- Frequency of turns and position changes
- Edema
- Venous thromboembolism prophylaxis
- Rest and sleep
- Endurance/cardiorespiratory status.

In the acute setting, the rehabilitation team can also provide:

- Psychological support to patient and/or family
- Educational programs on stroke, stroke prevention, and personal care
- Functional mobility skills assessment and exercises
  - Bed mobility
  - Transfers
  - Wheelchair or assistive device mobility.

Care in this setting is ideally directed by a physician with training and expertise in neurorehabilitation, and carried out by a team, with weekly meetings for case discussion. Therapy duration is usually 3 hours per day. However, recent animal and human research studies suggest that, for brain plasticity and subsequent improvements to occur, rehabilitation be task-specific, repetitive, and motivating to the patient. Thus, additional 'bedside' therapy, ideally provided by other hospital staff, provides additional practice attempts harnessing the potential plasticity of the brain thought to be available during the acute stage of recovery. The rehabilitation team will also make the recommendation for what type of post stroke rehabilitation should occur.

POST STROKE REHABILITATION

After the patient is medically stable and diagnostic evaluations are complete, rehabilitation becomes the focus of care. This phase of care can be conducted in either inpatient or outpatient settings. If your hospital does not have a rehabilitation unit, then it is very important to establish close relationships with one or more rehabilitation facilities so that patients can be transferred and task-specific, repetitive rehabilitation can be started in a timely fashion. Ideally, the transition in care from the acute stroke center to the rehabilitation site should be seamless. A rehabilitation clinical path can help assure that the transition goes well.

STROKE REHABILITATION OUTCOMES

Several factors may influence the specific outcome of an individual patient involved in a post stroke rehabilitation program. Potentially important factors may include:

- Type, distribution, pattern, and severity of physical impairment
- Cognitive, language, communication, and learning ability
- Number, type, and severity of comorbid medical conditions
- Depression or other psychological impairment
- Coping ability and style
- Nature and degree of family and other social supports
- Type and quality of specific rehabilitation training programs.

The strongest and most consistent predictor of discharge functional ability is admission functional ability.[3] The strongest predictors of adverse outcomes are coma at onset, persistent incontinence, poor cognitive function, severe hemiplegia, prior stroke, visuo-spatial neglect, cardiovascular disease, and large cerebral lesion.[4] It is important to note that, although hundreds of articles describe numerous predictors of outcome after stroke rehabilitation, it is difficult to apply these predictors to a particular patient given the heterogeneous nature of stroke and the impact that premorbid factors can have on outcome.

NEW APPROACHES TO MOTOR AND FUNCTIONAL TRAINING

Traditionally, stroke patients have been encouraged to use their less affected hands. This has been based on the premise that motor recovery in the more affected hand is not plausible and, thus, compensatory strategies (e.g. one-handed shoelace tying, writing with the less affected hand) should be taught. During compensatory training, the patient is encouraged to make use of residual abilities to develop new ways of achieving old goals, and perform routine tasks such as transferring. Reduced lengths of stay have also forced therapists to focus on compensatory strategies using the less affected limb. Additional motor training programs have consisted of positioning, passive and active range of motion exercises, and progressive resistance exercises.

TASK-SPECIFIC TRAINING APPROACHES

As noted earlier, numerous studies have shown that movement patterns and anatomical regions used more frequently become represented over larger cortical surface areas. Based on this finding in both animals and humans, a number of new, task-specific training regimens have been developed and are being tested as new approaches to rehabilitation.

Constraint-induced movement therapy

For decades it had been observed that individuals with neurologic insults, although capable of using their more affected limbs, often chose not to use them.[5,6] However, following success in early conditioned response studies,[7] researchers forced use of patients' more affected limbs by requiring sling wear on their less affected limbs during nearly all waking hours of a 2-week period. Following the intervention, patients demonstrated significant but small improvements in 19 of the 21 motor tasks on the Wolf Motor Function Test.[8] Subsequent researchers[9–11] have combined a restriction schedule identical to the one used by Wolf and colleagues with a 6-hour/day training protocol during which patients perform functional tasks using the more affected limb. Training sessions occur on all weekdays of the same 2-week period that restriction of the less affected limb occurs. The studies have shown that this 'constraint-induced movement therapy' (CIT) causes substantial increases in use and function of the more affected limb in chronic stroke patients (> 1 year post cerebrovascular accident (CVA)) and, more recently, in more subacute stroke cases.[12] Despite the attention that CIT has received, data from only one large chronic CVA CIT randomized controlled study have been reported,[11] and its methods and conclusions were criticized.[13]

Modified constraint-induced therapy: an outpatient, reimbursable alternative

Because of efficacy in pilot studies, a large, multicenter CIT trial is underway. However, even if efficacy is shown, considerable data suggest that CIT may be difficult to implement because of poor patient compliance. A recent survey[14] found that many stroke patients would not want to participate

Figure 9.1

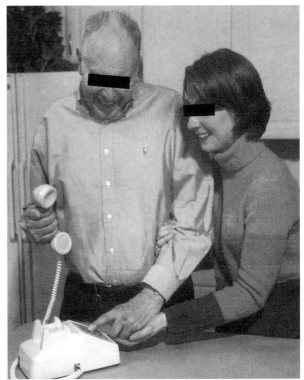

Patient participating in modified constraint-induced therapy with the guidance of his therapist

in CIT, and would prefer a therapy protocol lasting for more weeks with shorter activity sessions and/or fewer hours wearing the restrictive devices. Given CIT shortcomings, shorter forced use protocols have been developed.[15,16] The most notable example has been an outpatient therapy called 'modified constraint-induced therapy' (mCIT), which combines 30-minute activities of daily living (ADL) practice sessions with restriction of the unaffected arm 5 days/week for 5 hours/day, both during a 10-week period (Figure 9.1). Besides being reimbursable by most managed care programs, mCIT increases affected arm use and function in randomized, controlled studies with acute,[17] subacute (>3 months <12 months post stroke),[18,19] and chronic[20] stroke patients.

Following stroke, the size of the cortical representation of the more affected hand is known to decrease.[21–23] However, as stated earlier, in task-specific protocols like mCIT, in which the more affected limb is used in behaviorally relevant ways, the size of the cortical areas representing the limb increases.[24–27] As such, increased functional use of the affected arm via mCIT participation has been suggested to cause cortical reorganization.

Bilateral training

Imagine signing your first name on a chalkboard using your non-dominant hand at normal speed, but moving in the direction opposite to normal (the product should look like a mirror image of how your signature normally appears). Unless you have practiced, you are likely to have to think about this as you perform this task, and the movement outcome (your signature) is likely to be suboptimal. Now, attempt this same task again, but simultaneously write your name as you normally would using your dominant hand. You are likely to find that this combined, bilateral regimen is easier, and that the movement outcome is significantly better. More importantly, you will probably notice that the two hands appear to be 'locked' together.

As the above experiment shows, our limbs are indeed 'locked,' which has commonly been termed 'entrainment.' However, while the above experiment shows that the limbs are *spatially* entrained, studies have also shown that the limbs are *temporally* entrained. For example, it is very difficult to tap a constant rhythm with one hand while tapping as quickly as possible with the other. Similarly, research shows that individuals listening to an externally produced, constant rhythm (e.g. a metronome) tend to have difficulty tapping out a consistent but completely different rhythm.[28] It is believed that this entrainment effect is seen because a single neural mechanism controls spatial and temporal aspects of both limbs. The use of this single mechanism makes it difficult to 'beat the system' by simultaneously employing more than one movement pattern without considerable practice.

Following stroke, the above entrainment effect is retained. More importantly, research suggests that a particular patient who is unable to move the affected arm voluntarily by itself can often move the arm when bilateral practice strategies are employed. This is a critical discovery, as it means that patients who normally would be barely able to move their affected arms if a unilateral practice strategy was employed are often able to move the affected limb – and practice meaningfully – when bilateral training strategies are employed. Of course, bilateral training is also useful in relearning activities that are naturally bilateral (e.g. walking). And, bilateral training has also been shown to produce increased strength, range of motion, and performance of discrete unilateral and bilateral movement in the affected limbs of stroke patients.[29]

Bilateral training may also be optimal for stroke patients because they receive proprioceptive and visual feedback from the unaffected limb that they do not receive during unilateral practice in which only the affected limb is used. Indeed, when practicing bilaterally, a patient can use the unaffected extremity's neurologically intact afferent and efferent signals, and the look and feel of movement within that limb, to promote similar movement in the affected limb. For example, a stroke patient could simultaneously practice a reaching movement, such as reaching for a cup, with the affected and unaffected limb. This would provide sensory input, as the patient feels what it is like to reach for the cup in the unaffected limb. However, the visual input of seeing the unaffected arm reach for the cup may also provide a model with which the patient can better move the affected limb and become more successful.

Interestingly, bilateral training is also inherent in walking, which is thought to be a primary reason why the lower extremity tends to recover more rapidly than the upper extremity. However, despite the fact that proprioceptive training of the hemiparetic lower extremity is inherent during ambulation (i.e. the 'feel' of walking), the visual feedback needed to implement true bilateral training is *not* as available as it is with the upper extremity, as the subject is not looking down to check feet position, hip angle, and so on, as this puts the patient at risk for falls. Clinicians have somewhat solved this limited visual feedback by placing a mirror at the end of a treadmill and having the patient walk 'towards' the mirror. If improved function is realized through increased feedback and integration of the lower extremities, how can the clinical setting be altered to approximate the same conditions for the upper extremities?

Current models of bilateral training in stroke

Bilateral arm training with rhythmic auditory cueing (BATRAC) uses a robot to deliver controlled, bilateral, rhythmic movements to the upper limbs and has been shown to be effective. Although the BATRAC serves as a useful tool to study bilateral training under optimal conditions, most therapy clinics do not have robotic arms and cannot afford to invest in these types of strategies.

At the University of Cincinnati, we have used the NuStep to administer bilateral training for the arms

Figure 9.2

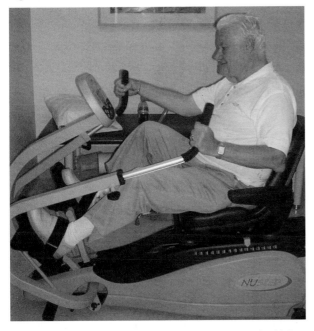

Patient participating in bilateral, reciprocal training using the NuStep

and legs. As shown in Figure 9.2, the NuStep is a commonly available machine that has traditionally been used to rehabilitate and/or strengthen geriatric patients. However, the NuStep also allows the patient to oppositionally, bilaterally practice with both legs and both arms simultaneously. Importantly, whereas many approaches to affected limb function in stroke require intense supervised practice, specialized training, and/or additional personnel, the NuStep is easy to use, requires minimal supervision, and widespread application can be quickly realized. The device has the advantage that the patient can engage in bilateral practice that simulates walking while remaining seated.

Pilot data suggest that the NuStep is a promising clinically practical approach to improving balance and ambulation in stroke patients, even many years after injury. Importantly, the resistance on the device can be adjusted, resulting in marked improvement in cardiovascular conditioning in most of our subjects. Currently, we are investigating the use of an auditory component (e.g. a metronome), as auditory cueing is believed to increase learning of naturally rhythmic behaviors such as walking.

ELECTRICAL STIMULATION

Despite growing evidence suggesting that motor relearning after stroke is activity-dependent, large

segments of the population of stroke survivors are not able to take part in such strategies due to the severity of their hemiparesis and/or growing resource limitations of the evolving health care environment. Cyclic neuromuscular electrical stimulation (NMES) involves stimulation applied to the affected muscle(s) to elicit muscle contraction(s). It is presumed that the afferent input improves motor control with repeated use. Several studies have shown increased affected arm function following cyclic surface NMES use.[30] However, cyclic surface NMES therapy may be suboptimal because patients are not responsible for volitionally activating their muscles (i.e. their participation is passive).

Given that repeated, *volitional*, affected limb use facilitates improved function, it would seem advantageous to use a device focused on that type of activity. Surface electromyography (EMG)-triggered neuromuscular stimulation (ETMS) incorporates concepts of repeated limb use, biofeedback, and electrical stimulation. When using ETMS, the patient attempts to activate the affected musculature (for the purposes of this discussion, the affected extensors). If the intended muscles are activated such that a pre-set threshold is reached (as detected by EMG in the device), the musculature will be electrically stimulated by the device and full extension is realized. If the threshold is not reached, the threshold is automatically lowered, and the patient tries again. Thus, the patient is provided with biofeedback that 'reteaches' active muscle contraction through the reward of stimulation. ETMS appears to restore more affected wrist movement in both subacute and chronic stroke patients.[31–33]

A new electrical stimulation approach is testing a hand orthosis that provides synchronized activation of finger and wrist flexors and extensors during practice of functional, valued ADLs.[34,35] The device, called the 'Handmaster,' can be self-administered in the home, making it more accessible to a larger number of stroke patients than traditional modalities, which typically require therapist supervision in a structured environment. The device is used during performance of valued ADLs, which overcomes a shortcoming of passive, electrical stimulation modalities. The device is depicted in Figure 9.3.

CONCLUSION

There is an increasing prevalence of stroke survivors in the United States, due to improved acute therapies

Figure 9.3

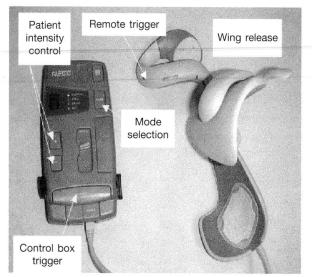

(a)

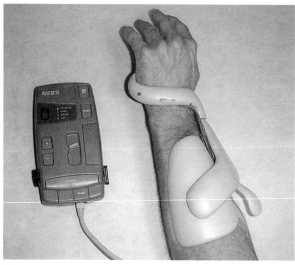

(b)

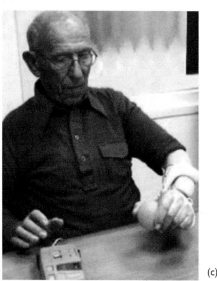

(c)

(a) The H-200 electrical stimulation orthosis; (b and c) a stroke patient using the H-200 during a functional grasp–release task

and better management of stroke comorbidities. Because of the increased survival rate, stroke rehabilitation will play an even greater role in returning patients to a normal level of function and quality of life. Ideally, stroke rehabilitation emphasizes a team approach that, while physiatrist-directed, also includes input from therapy staff, neuropsychologists, social workers and, most importantly, the patient's family and the patient. Stroke caregivers and clinicians should remember that meaningful recovery can occur months and even years after stroke; task-specific repetitive practice and an open-minded clinician are fundamental to this continued recovery process.

REFERENCES

1. Duncan PW, Zorowitz R, Bates B et al. Management of Adult Stroke Rehabilitation Care: a clinical practice guideline. Stroke 2005; 36(9): e100–43.
2. Roth EJ, Harvey RL. Rehabilitation of stroke syndromes. In Braddom RL (ed): Physical Medicine and Rehabilitation. Philadelphia: WB Saunders, 2000, pp 1117–63.
3. Jongbloed L. Prediction of function after stroke: a critical review. Stroke 1986; 17(4): 765–76.
4. Dombovy ML, Sandok BA, Basford JR. Rehabilitation for stroke: a review. Stroke 1986; 17(3): 363–9.
5. Tower SS. Pyramidal lesions in the monkey. Brain 1940; 63: 36–90.
6. Lashley KS. Studies of cerebral function in learning: the retention of motor areas in primates. Arch Neurol Psychiatry 1924; 12: 249–76.
7. Halberstam JL, Zaretsky HH, Brucker BS, Guttman AR. Avoidance conditioning of motor responses in elderly brain-damaged patients. Arch Phys Med Rehabil 1971; 52(7): 318–27 passim.
8. Wolf SL, Lecraw DE, Barton LA, Jann BB. Forced use of hemiplegic upper extremities to reverse the effect of learned nonuse among chronic stroke and head-injured patients. Exp Neurol 1989; 104(2): 125–32.
9. Taub E, Miller NE, Novack TA et al. Technique to improve chronic motor deficit after stroke. Arch Phys Med Rehabil 1993; 74(4): 347–54.
10. Miltner WH, Bauder H, Sommer M, Dettmers C, Taub E. Effects of constraint-induced movement therapy on patients with chronic motor deficits after stroke: a replication. Stroke 1999; 30(3): 586–92.
11. van der Lee JH, Wagenaar RC, Lankhorst GJ,

Vogelaar TW, Deville WL, Bouter LM. Forced use of the upper extremity in chronic stroke patients: results from a single-blind randomized clinical trial. Stroke 1999; 30(11): 2369–75.

12. Blanton S, Wolf SL. An application of upper-extremity constraint-induced movement therapy in a patient with subacute stroke. Phys Ther 1999; 79(9): 847–53.

13. Taub E. Constraint-induced movement therapy and massed practice. Stroke 2000; 31(4): 986–8.

14. Page SJ, Levine P, Sisto S, Bond Q, Johnston MV. Stroke patients' and therapists' opinions of constraint-induced movement therapy. Clin Rehabil 2002; 16(1): 55–60.

15. Sterr A, Elbert T, Berthold I, Kolbel S, Rockstroh B, Taub E. Longer versus shorter daily constraint-induced movement therapy of chronic hemiparesis: an exploratory study. Arch Phys Med Rehabil 2002; 83(10): 1374–7.

16. Pierce SR, Gallagher KG, Schaumburg SW, Gershkoff AM, Gaughan JP, Shutter L. Home forced use in an outpatient rehabilitation program for adults with hemiplegia: a pilot study. Neurorehabil Neural Repair 2003; 17(4): 214–19.

17. Page SJ, Levine P, Leonard AC. Modified constraint-induced therapy in acute stroke: a randomized controlled pilot study. Neurorehabil Neural Repair 2005; 19(1): 27–32.

18. Page SJ, Sisto SA, Levine P, Johnston MV, Hughes M. Modified constraint induced therapy: a randomized feasibility and efficacy study. J Rehabil Res Dev 2001; 38(5): 583–90.

19. Page SJ, Sisto S, Johnston MV, Levine P. Modified constraint-induced therapy after subacute stroke: a preliminary study. Neurorehabil Neural Repair 2002; 16(3): 290–5.

20. Page SJ, Gater DR, Bach-Y-Rita P. Reconsidering the motor recovery plateau in stroke rehabilitation. Arch Phys Med Rehabil 2004; 85(8): 1377–81.

21. Cicinelli P, Traversa R, Rossini PM. Post-stroke reorganization of brain motor output to the hand: a 2–4 month follow-up with focal magnetic transcranial stimulation. Electroencephalogr Clin Neurophysiol 1997; 105(6): 438–50.

22. Traversa R, Cicinelli P, Bassi A, Rossini PM, Bernardi G. Mapping of motor cortical reorganization after stroke. A brain stimulation study with focal magnetic pulses. Stroke 1997; 28(1): 110–17.

23. Nudo RJ, Milliken GW, Jenkins WM, Merzenich MM. Use-dependent alterations of movement repre-sentations in primary motor cortex of adult squirrel monkeys. J Neurosci 1996; 16(2): 785–807.

24. Classen J, Liepert J, Wise SP, Hallett M, Cohen LG. Rapid plasticity of human cortical movement repre-sentation induced by practice. J Neurophysiol 1998; 79(2): 1117–23.

25. Liepert J, Terborg C, Weiller C. Motor plasticity induced by synchronized thumb and foot movements. Exp Brain Res 1999; 125(4): 435–9.

26. Elbert T, Pantev C, Wienbruch C, Rockstroh B, Taub E. Increased cortical representation of the fingers of the left hand in string players. Science 1995; 270(5234): 305–7.

27. Sterr A, Muller MM, Elbert T, Rockstroh B, Pantev C, Taub E. Changed perceptions in Braille readers. Nature 1998; 391(6663): 134–5.

28. Klapp ST, Hill MD, Tyier JG, Martin ZE, Jagacinski RJ, Jones MR. On marching to two different drummers: perceptual aspects of the difficulties. J Exp Psychol Hum Percept Perform 1985; 11(6): 814–27.

29. Whitall J, McCombe Waller S, Silver KH, Macko RF. Repetitive bilateral arm training with rhythmic auditory cueing improves motor function in chronic hemiparetic stroke. Stroke 2000; 31(10): 2390–5.

30. Liberson WT, Holmquest HJ, Scot D, Dow M. Functional electrotherapy: stimulation of the peroneal nerve synchronized with the swing phase of the gait of hemiplegic patients. Arch Phys Med Rehabil 1961; 42: 101–5.

31. Chae J, Bethoux F, Bohine T, Dobos L, Davis T, Friedl A. Neuromuscular stimulation for upper extremity motor and functional recovery in acute hemiplegia. Stroke 1998; 29(5): 975–9.

32. Powell J, Pandyan AD, Granat M, Cameron M, Stott DJ. Electrical stimulation of wrist extensors in poststroke hemiplegia. Stroke 1999; 30(7): 1384–9.

33. Sonde L, Gip C, Fernaeus SE, Nilsson CG, Viitanen M. Stimulation with low frequency (1.7 Hz) transcu-taneous electric nerve stimulation (low-tens) increases motor function of the post-stroke paretic arm. Scand J Rehabil Med 1998; 30(2): 95–9.

34. Alon G, Sunnerhagen KS, Geurts AC, Ohry A. A home-based, self-administered stimulation program to improve selected hand functions of chronic stroke. NeuroRehabilitation 2003; 18(3): 215–25.

35. McBride AG, Ring KH. Improving selected hand functions using non-invasive neuroprosthesis in persons with chronic stroke. J Stroke Cerebrovasc Dis 2002; 11(2): 99–106.

Appendix

Clinical scales and tools

One of the most effective ways to assure efficient quality care in the stroke center is to use standardized tools. Some of these, such as clinical pathways and order sets, will be specific to your stroke center and some will be scales and tools that are used uniformly across all centers. The latter are useful for comparing your performance and outcomes with other centers. There is good evidence that when standardized order tools are utilized, care improves.[1] This section includes some of the more commonly used clinical scales. They can be downloaded from strokecenter.org/trials/scales/indes. There are also sample tools and educational materials developed by the Saint Luke's Hospital Stroke Team.

PREHOSPITAL CLINICAL ASSESSMENT TOOLS

Two prehospital tools are included here. Both have been used very effectively by emergency medical providers in accurately diagnosing stroke prior to arrival at the hospital. The Cincinnati Stroke Scale is also a useful tool for public education and awareness of stroke symptoms.

CINCINNATI PREHOSPITAL STROKE SCALE

Facial droop
    Normal: Both sides of face move equally
    Abnormal: One side of face does not move at all

Arm drift
    Normal: Both arms move equally or not at all
    Abnormal: One arm drifts compared to the other

Speech
    Normal: Patient uses correct words with no slurring
    Abnormal: Slurred or inappropriate words or mute

REFERENCE

Kothari RU, Pancioli A, Liu T, Brott T, Broderick J. Cincinnati Prehospital Stroke Scale: reproducibility and validity. Ann Emerg Med 1999; 33: 373–8.

Provided by the Internet Stroke Center – www.strokecenter.org

---

LOS ANGELES PREHOSPITAL STROKE SCREEN (LAPSS)

Patient Name: _____

Rater Name: _____

Date: _____

Screening Criteria	Yes	No
4. Age over 45 years	____	____
5. No prior history of seizure disorder	____	____
6. New onset of neurologic symptoms in last 24 hours	____	____
7. Patient was ambulatory at baseline (prior to event)	____	____
8. Blood glucose between 60 and 400	____	____

9. Exam: *look for obvious asymmetry*

	Normal	Right	Left
Facial smile/grimace:	☐	☐ Droop	☐ Droop
Grip:	☐	☐ Weak Grip ☐ No Grip	☐ Weak Grip ☐ No Grip
Arm weakness:	☐	☐ Drifts Down ☐ Falls Rapidly	☐ Drifts Down ☐ Falls Rapidly

Based on exam, patient has only unilateral (and not bilateral) weakness: Yes ☐ No ☐

10. If Yes (or unknown) to all items above LAPSS screening criteria met: Yes ☐ No ☐

11. If LAPSS criteria for stroke met, call receiving hospital with "CODE STROKE", if not then return to the appropriate treatment protocol. (Note: the patient may still be experiencing a stroke even if LAPSS criteria are not met.)

REFERENCE

Kidwell CS, Starkman S, Eckstein M, Weems K, Saver JL. Identifying stroke in the field. Prospective validation of the Los Angeles prehospital stroke screen (LAPSS). Stroke 2000; 31: 71–6.

Provided by the Internet Stroke Center – www.strokecenter.org

EMERGENCY DEPARTMENT TOOLS

If acute stroke intervention is going to be provided then standardized efficient care in the emergency department (ED) is essential. It is helpful for comprehensive centers to provide information to primary centers regarding treatment options and the transfer process. Each ED should have a flowsheet for summarizing the important aspects of acute stroke treatment.

Saint Luke's Hospital of Kansas City
SAINT LUKE'S-SHAWNEE MISSION HEALTH SYSTEM

Emergency Department Neurology Clinical Path

NIH STROKE SCALE Category	Description/Score	Adm NIH	Dsch NIH
1a. Level of Consciousness (If patient scores either 2 or 3 in this section of the neuro check, proceed to the Glasgow Coma Scale)	Alert – 0 / Drowsy – 1 / Stuporous – 2 / Coma – 3		
1b. LOC Questions (Month, Age)	Answers Both Correctly – 0 / Answers One Correctly – 1 / Incorrect – 2		
1c. LOC Commands (Open, close eyes, make fist, let go)	Obeys Both Correctly – 0 / Obeys One Correctly – 1 / Performs neither task – 2		
2. Best Gaze (Eyes open-patient follows examiner's fingers/face)	Normal – 0 / Partial Gaze Palsy – 1 / Forced Deviation – 2		
3. Visual (Introduce visual stimulus (or threat) to patient's visual field quadrants)	No Visual Loss – 0 / Partial Hemianopia – 1 / Complete Hemianopia – 2 / Bilateral Hemianopia – 3		
4. Facial Palsy (Show teeth, raise eyebrows, and squeezes eyes shut)	Normal – 0 / Minor paralysis – 1 / Partial paralysis – 2 / Complete paralysis – 3		
5a. Motor Left Arm (Elevate extremity to 90° and score drift/movement) (Do not add amputation score in final NIH score)	No Drift – 0 / Drift – 1 / Can't Resist Gravity – 2 / No Effort Against Gravity – 3 / No Movement – 4 / Amputation, Joint Fusion – UN		
5b. Motor Right Arm (Elevate extremity to 90° and score drift/movement) (Do not add amputation score in final NIH score)	No Drift – 0 / Drift – 1 / Can't Resist Gravity – 2 / No Effort Against Gravity – 3 / No Movement – 4 / Amputation, Joint Fusion – UN		
6a. Motor Left Leg (Elevate extremity to 90° and score drift/movement) (Do not add amputation score in final NIH score)	No Drift – 0 / Drift – 1 / Can't Resist Gravity – 2 / No Effort Against Gravity – 3 / No Movement – 4 / Amputation, Joint Fusion – UN		
6b. Motor Right Leg (Elevate extremity to 90° and score drift/movement) (Do not add amputation score in final NIH score)	No Drift – 0 / Drift – 1 / Can't Resist Gravity – 2 / No Effort Against Gravity – 3 / No Movement – 4 / Amputation, Joint Fusion – UN		
7. Limb Ataxia	Absent – 0 / Present In One Limb – 1 / Present In Two Limbs – 2		
8. Sensory (Pinprick to face, arm, trunk and leg)	Normal – 0 / Partial Loss – 1 / Severe Loss – 2		
9. Best Language (Name items, describe a picture, read sentence)	No Aphasia – 0 / Mild to Moderate Aphasia – 1 / Severe Aphasia – 2 / Mute – 3		
10. Dysarthria (Evaluate Speech Clarity)	Normal Articulation – 0 / Mild to Mod Dysarthria – 1 / Near to Unintelligible – 2 / Intubated/Other Barrier – UN		
11. Extinction and Inattention (Use information from prior testing to identify neglect)	No Neglect – 0 / Partial Neglect – 1 / Profound Neglect – 2		
	TOTAL		

PATIENT LABEL

ASSESSMENT DIAGNOSTICS TREATMENT PATIENT TEACHING

Date:

Diagnosis:
- [ ] Ischemic Stroke
- [ ] Hemorrhagic Stroke
- [ ] TIA
- [ ] Other_____

- [ ] Vitals q1°
- [ ] Baseline NIHSS
- [ ] GCS if LOC ≥ 2 q1°
- [ ] Est. Weight_____ lbs/kg
- [ ] Telemetry

- [ ] Stroke Panel (Lytes, Glucose, Creatine, CBC, Coag Screen)
- [ ] EKG
- [ ] Baseline O2 Sat_____%
- [ ] PBG_____
  (Notify Dr. if <70 or >150)

(CT Results)
- [ ] Negative / Nothing Acute
- [ ] Hemorrhage
- [ ] New Ischemic Stroke
- [ ] Other

- [ ] Initiate Acute Stroke Standing Orders
- [ ] ASA SUPP OR P.O. NPO
- [ ] Acetaminophen 325 mg supp if T>99
- [ ] BP Protocol
  - Ischemic: target BP 185/100
  - Hemorrhagic: target BP 140/80
  - No Sublinguinal Nifedipine
- [ ] Research Study Drug_____
- [ ] O2 2-4L if O2 sat <90
- [ ] Weight Based Heparin Orders
Bolus_____

Time Given [:]
Unit/Hr_____

- [ ] Give family hospital Data Base and instruct on section to begin completing
- [ ] Need for diagnostic tests discussed with patient/family.

Time patient admitted to [:]
Room #_____

Transfer from other facility? [ ] Yes [ ] No
Other Facility Triage Time [:]

Facility_____

TPA Given? [ ] Yes [ ] No
If Yes, dosage & Time TPA started [:]

[ ] 0.6 mgm/kg   [ ] 0.9 mgm/kg

SLHED Triage [:]
Stroke Onset [:]

TIME

NO | YES   ONSET ≤ 5 HRS: Triage   Urgent
- → Seen by ED Physician: [:]
- → Neuro Evaluation: (phone or in person) [:]
- → CT Head Scan done: [:]
- → TPA CHECKLIST COMPLETE [ ]
- → Thrombolytic started: [:]

(check one)
- [ ] IV
- [ ] INTRA-ARTERIAL
- [ ] IV & INTRA-ARTERIAL

Total dose_____mg

Reason excluded from thrombolysis: (circle one)
→ TIME   BP   OTHER:_____

TPA CHECKLIST
- [ ] Onset ≤ 3 Hours (IV)
- [ ] Onset ≤ 6 Hours (IA)
- [ ] No Hemorrhage on CT Scan
- [ ] BP < 185/110
- [ ] Platelets > 100,000
- [ ] INR < 1.5
- [ ] Protime < 15 Sec.
- [ ] Glucose > 50 < 400
- [ ] No recent major surgery, trauma, stroke, LP, non-compressible arterial puncture, active internal bleeding
- [ ] If foley needed, insert before thrombolytic
- [ ] Consent signed

Initial	SIGNATURE	Initial	SIGNATURE

Symbol Key
"✓" in a ☐ box means item was completed
"O" in a ☐ box indicates the items was not pertinent

Mid America Brain and Stroke Institute
SAINT LUKE'S HOSPITAL

Emergency Department
Neurology Clinical Path

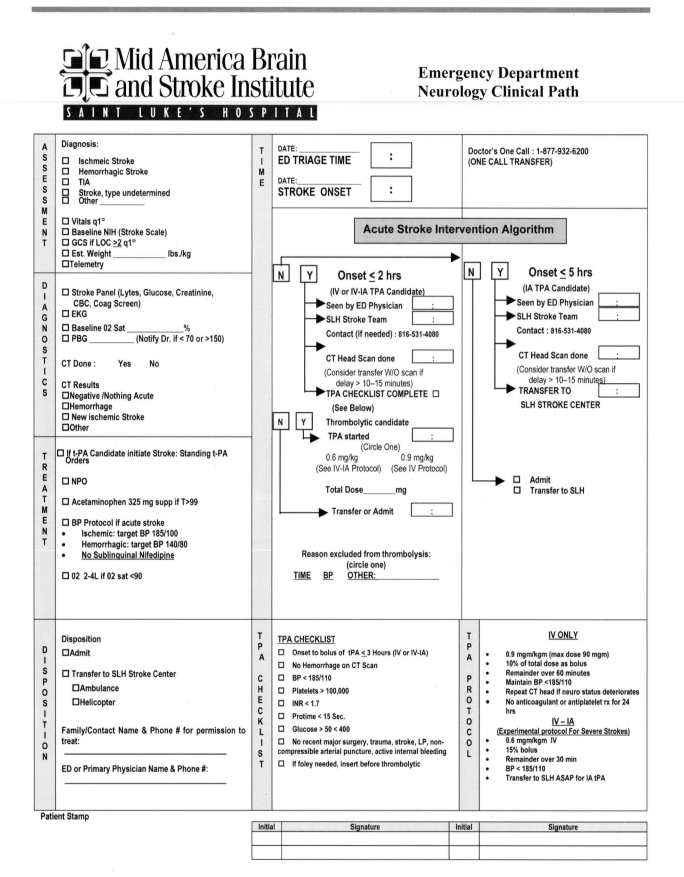

ASSESSMENT

Diagnosis:
- ☐ Ischmeic Stroke
- ☐ Hemorrhagic Stroke
- ☐ TIA
- ☐ Stroke, type undetermined
- ☐ Other _____

- ☐ Vitals q1°
- ☐ Baseline NIH (Stroke Scale)
- ☐ GCS if LOC >2 q1°
- ☐ Est. Weight _____ lbs./kg
- ☐ Telemetry

DIAGNOSTICS

- ☐ Stroke Panel (Lytes, Glucose, Creatinine, CBC, Coag Screen)
- ☐ EKG
- ☐ Baseline 02 Sat _____ %
- ☐ PBG _____ (Notify Dr. if < 70 or >150)

CT Done :   Yes   No

CT Results
- ☐ Negative /Nothing Acute
- ☐ Hemorrhage
- ☐ New ischemic Stroke
- ☐ Other

TREATMENT

- ☐ If t-PA Candidate initiate Stroke: Standing t-PA Orders
- ☐ NPO
- ☐ Acetaminophen 325 mg supp if T>99
- ☐ BP Protocol if acute stroke
  - Ischemic: target BP 185/100
  - Hemorrhagic: target BP 140/80
  - No Sublinquinal Nifedipine
- ☐ 02 2-4L if 02 sat <90

TIME

DATE: _____
ED TRIAGE TIME   :

DATE: _____
STROKE ONSET   :

Doctor's One Call : 1-877-932-6200
(ONE CALL TRANSFER)

Acute Stroke Intervention Algorithm

N Y   **Onset ≤ 2 hrs**
(IV or IV-IA TPA Candidate)
→ Seen by ED Physician   :
→ SLH Stroke Team   :
Contact (if needed) : 816-531-4080

→ CT Head Scan done   :
(Consider transfer W/O scan if delay > 10–15 minutes)
→ TPA CHECKLIST COMPLETE ☐
(See Below)

N Y   Thrombolytic candidate
→ TPA started   :
(Circle One)
0.6 mg/kg   0.9 mg/kg
(See IV-IA Protocol)   (See IV Protocol)

Total Dose_____mg

→ Transfer or Admit   :

Reason excluded from thrombolysis:
(circle one)
TIME   BP   OTHER: _____

N Y   **Onset ≤ 5 hrs**
(IA TPA Candidate)
→ Seen by ED Physician   :
→ SLH Stroke Team   :
Contact : 816-531-4080

CT Head Scan done   :
(Consider transfer W/O scan if delay > 10–15 minutes)
→ TRANSFER TO   :
SLH STROKE CENTER

→ ☐ Admit
   ☐ Transfer to SLH

DISPOSITION

Disposition
- ☐ Admit
- ☐ Transfer to SLH Stroke Center
  - ☐ Ambulance
  - ☐ Helicopter

Family/Contact Name & Phone # for permission to treat:
_____

ED or Primary Physician Name & Phone #:
_____

TPA CHECKLIST

TPA CHECKLIST
- ☐ Onset to bolus of tPA ≤ 3 Hours (IV or IV-IA)
- ☐ No Hemorrhage on CT Scan
- ☐ BP < 185/110
- ☐ Platelets > 100,000
- ☐ INR < 1.7
- ☐ Protime < 15 Sec.
- ☐ Glucose > 50 < 400
- ☐ No recent major surgery, trauma, stroke, LP, non-compressible arterial puncture, active internal bleeding
- ☐ If foley needed, insert before thrombolytic

TPA PROTOCOL

IV ONLY
- 0.9 mgm/kgm (max dose 90 mgm)
- 10% of total dose as bolus
- Remainder over 60 minutes
- Maintain BP <185/110
- Repeat CT head if neuro status deteriorates
- No anticoagulant or antiplatelet rx for 24 hrs

IV – IA
(Experimental protocol For Severe Strokes)
- 0.6 mgm/kgm IV
- 15% bolus
- Remainder over 30 min
- BP < 185/110
- Transfer to SLH ASAP for IA tPA

Patient Stamp

Initial	Signature	Initial	Signature

MID AMERICA BRAIN AND STROKE INSTITUTE
SAINT LUKE'S HOSPITAL

CURRENT OPTIONS FOR ACUTE STROKE INTERVENTION

1. **Patient presenting within <u>3 hours</u> of symptom onset who meets criteria for treatment with IV (intravenous) tPA.**

   - Standard (FDA approved, 1996) IV tPA at 0.9 mgm/kgm (max dose = 90 mgm); 10% bolus, the rest over 1 hour. Blood pressure to be 185/110 or lower at the time of treatment and maintained at <180/105 or lower after treatment. No anticoagulants or antiplatelets for 24 hours. No hemorrhage on CT head scan. No special consent needed.
   - For more severe strokes, consider the experimental protocol: give IV tPA 0.6 mgm/kgm 15% bolus, the rest over 30 minutes, followed by intra-arterial (IA) tPA. The initial IV treatment must be started within 3 hours of onset of symptoms, can be given at the local ED and the patient can come to the Saint Luke's Hospital Mid America Brain and Stroke Institute by helicopter or ambulance for the therapy which must begin in the 5 hours after symptom onset. We will obtain consent when the patient arrives. No special consent required for the IV administration. Same CT and BP requirements.

2. **Patient presenting <u>after 3 hours but within 6</u> hours of symptom onset who meets criteria for treatment with IA tPA.**

   - Patient can have IA tPA as long as the procedure is started by 6 hours after onset. This is usually reserved for severe strokes and is experimental. We have had excellent outcomes with this approach.

3. **Patient presenting within <u>8 hours</u> of symptoms onset.**

   - Patient can be treated with the MERCI clot retrieval device that can remove the clot from the middle cerebral, basilar or internal carotid arteries.
   - This procedure can be combined with IV and/or IA tPA.
   - In August 2004 FDA approved this catheter for clot retrieval.

The Mid America Brain and Stroke Team Neurologists and Interventional Neuroradiologists are available 24/7. The best access number is the **Doctors' One Call number at 816-932-6200**. Saint Luke's is NEVER on diversion for stroke.

SAINT LUKE'S HOSPITAL
KANSAS CITY, MISSOURI

PHYSICIAN'S PLANS (ORDERS)

USE BALL POINT PEN – PRESS FIRMLY

DATE	TIME	PROB NO.	ANOTHER BRAND OF DRUG IDENTICAL IN FORM AND CONTENT MAY BE DISPENSED UNLESS CHECKED. ☐
			STROKE: Standing Tissue Plasminogen Activase (t-PA) Orders
		1.	Admit to ED Diagnosis Stroke
		2.	Stat Labs (CBC with platelets, Electrolyte, Creatinine, Glucose, PTT, PT, INR)
		3.	Stat EKG
		4.	Stat CT of head – non contrast
		5.	Establish exact onset time of symptoms – Notify Saint Luke's Doctors' One Call (877-932-6200) to discuss
			Treatment options with neurologists and transfer options with Doctors' One Call nurse.
		6.	Monitor oxygenation, place on O_2 per nasal cannula if O_2 sat < 94
		7.	IV x 2 large bore; one in each arm
			a. NS at 50 cc/hour
			b. Saline lock second IV and use for possible t-PA infusion
		8.	Weight (approximate) _____ lbs _____ kgs
		9.	If patient a candidate for IV t-PA see Saint Luke's ED Flow Sheet for inclusion/exclusion criteria
		10.	Monitor BP frequently if t-PA candidate; maintain BP < 185/110
			a. If BP > 185/110, give Labetalol 10 mg IV over 1-2 minutes; can be repeated q 15 minutes.
			b. Do not exceed 300 mg. If unable to lower BP < 185/110 patient is not a t-PA candidate
		11.	Insert foley catheter if needed prior to administering of IV t-PA
		12.	**STANDARD IV t-PA Dosing**
			a. 0.9 mgm/kgm (max dose 90 mgm) Total IV t-PA _____ mg
			b. Give 10% of total dose as IV bolus. IV bolus _____ mg
			c. Infuse remainder t-PA over 60 minutes per IV pump. Infusion amount _____ mg
			d. Maintain BP < 185/110
			e. Repeat CT head if neuro status deteriorates
			f. No anticoagulant or antiplatelet treatment for 24 hours
		13.	**IV – IA t-PA Thrombolysis (Experimental protocol for Severe Strokes)**
			a. 0.6 mgm/kg IV bolus Total IV t-PA _____ mg
			b. Give 15% of total dose as IV bolus. IV bolus _____ mg
			c. Infuse remainder t-PA over 30 minutes per IV pump Infusion amount _____ mg
			d. Maintain BP < 185/110
			e. Transfer to Saint Luke's ASAP for IA t-PA (Doctors' One Nurse will assist with triage per Life Flight)
			Physician Signature/Date: _____

0.6 mg/kg tPA Dosing Chart
(total IV dose = 0.6 mg/kg, 15% of dose given as bolus, 85% as infusion. Maximum dose is 60 mg)

Wt (lb)	Wt (kg)	Total IV dose	15% Bolus	85% Infusion	Wt (lb)	Wt (kg)	Total IV dose	15% Bolus	85% Infusion
88	40.0	24.0	3.6	20.4	156	70.9	42.5	6.4	36.2
89	40.5	24.3	3.6	20.6	157	71.4	42.8	6.4	36.4
90	40.9	24.5	3.7	20.9	158	71.8	43.1	6.5	36.6
91	41.4	24.8	3.7	21.1	159	72.3	43.4	6.5	36.9
92	41.8	25.1	3.8	21.3	160	72.7	43.6	6.5	37.1
93	42.3	25.4	3.8	21.6	161	73.2	43.9	6.6	37.3
94	42.7	25.6	3.8	21.8	162	73.6	44.2	6.6	37.6
95	43.2	25.9	3.9	22.0	163	74.1	44.5	6.7	37.8
96	43.6	26.2	3.9	22.3	164	74.5	44.7	6.7	38.0
97	44.1	26.5	4.0	22.5	165	75.0	45.0	6.8	38.3
98	44.5	26.7	4.0	22.7	166	75.5	45.3	6.8	38.5
99	45.0	27.0	4.1	23.0	167	75.9	45.5	6.8	38.7
100	45.5	27.3	4.1	23.2	168	76.4	45.8	6.9	38.9
101	45.9	27.5	4.1	23.4	169	76.8	46.1	6.9	39.2
102	46.4	27.8	4.2	23.6	170	77.3	46.4	7.0	39.4
103	46.8	28.1	4.2	23.9	171	77.7	46.6	7.0	39.6
104	47.3	28.4	4.3	24.1	172	78.2	46.9	7.0	39.9
105	47.7	28.6	4.3	24.3	173	78.6	47.2	7.1	40.1
106	48.2	28.9	4.3	24.6	174	79.1	47.5	7.1	40.3
107	48.6	29.2	4.4	24.8	175	79.5	47.7	7.2	40.6
108	49.1	29.5	4.4	25.0	176	80.0	48.0	7.2	40.8
109	49.5	29.7	4.5	25.3	177	80.5	48.3	7.2	41.0
110	50.0	30.0	4.5	25.5	178	80.9	48.5	7.3	41.3
111	50.5	30.3	4.5	25.7	179	81.4	48.8	7.3	41.5
112	50.9	30.5	4.6	26.0	180	81.8	49.1	7.4	41.7
113	51.4	30.8	4.6	26.2	181	82.3	49.4	7.4	42.0
114	51.8	31.1	4.7	26.4	182	82.7	49.6	7.4	42.2
115	52.3	31.4	4.7	26.7	183	83.2	49.9	7.5	42.4
116	52.7	31.6	4.7	26.9	184	83.6	50.2	7.5	42.7
117	53.2	31.9	4.8	27.1	185	84.1	50.5	7.6	42.9
118	53.6	32.2	4.8	27.4	186	84.5	50.7	7.6	43.1
119	54.1	32.5	4.9	27.6	187	85.0	51.0	7.7	43.4
120	54.5	32.7	4.9	27.8	188	85.5	51.3	7.7	43.6
121	55.0	33.0	5.0	28.1	189	85.9	51.5	7.7	43.8
122	55.5	33.3	5.0	28.3	190	86.4	51.8	7.8	44.0
123	55.9	33.5	5.0	28.5	191	86.8	52.1	7.8	44.3
124	56.4	33.8	5.1	28.7	192	87.3	52.4	7.9	44.5
125	56.8	34.1	5.1	29.0	193	87.7	52.6	7.9	44.7
126	57.3	34.4	5.2	29.2	194	88.2	52.9	7.9	45.0
127	57.7	34.6	5.2	29.4	195	88.6	53.2	8.0	45.2
128	58.2	34.9	5.2	29.7	196	89.1	53.5	8.0	45.4
129	58.6	35.2	5.3	29.9	197	89.5	53.7	8.1	45.7
130	59.1	35.5	5.3	30.1	198	90.0	54.0	8.1	45.9
131	59.5	35.7	5.4	30.4	199	90.5	54.3	8.1	46.1
132	60.0	36.0	5.4	30.6	200	90.9	54.5	8.2	46.4
133	60.5	36.3	5.4	30.8	201	91.4	54.8	8.2	46.6
134	60.9	36.5	5.5	31.1	202	91.8	55.1	8.3	46.8
135	61.4	36.8	5.5	31.3	203	92.3	55.4	8.3	47.1
136	61.8	37.1	5.6	31.5	204	92.7	55.6	8.3	47.3
137	62.3	37.4	5.6	31.8	205	93.2	55.9	8.4	47.5
138	62.7	37.6	5.6	32.0	206	93.6	56.2	8.4	47.8
139	63.2	37.9	5.7	32.2	207	94.1	56.5	8.5	48.0
140	63.6	38.2	5.7	32.5	208	94.5	56.7	8.5	48.2
141	64.1	38.5	5.8	32.7	209	95.0	57.0	8.6	48.5
142	64.5	38.7	5.8	32.9	210	95.5	57.3	8.6	48.7
143	65.0	39.0	5.9	33.2	211	95.9	57.5	8.6	48.9
144	65.5	39.3	5.9	33.4	212	96.4	57.8	8.7	49.1
145	65.9	39.5	5.9	33.6	213	96.8	58.1	8.7	49.4
146	66.4	39.8	6.0	33.8	214	97.3	58.4	8.8	49.6
147	66.8	40.1	6.0	34.1	215	97.7	58.6	8.8	49.8
148	67.3	40.4	6.1	34.3	216	98.2	58.9	8.8	50.1
149	67.7	40.6	6.1	34.5	217	98.6	59.2	8.9	50.3
150	68.2	40.9	6.1	34.8	218	99.1	59.5	8.9	50.5
151	68.6	41.2	6.2	35.0	219	99.5	59.7	9.0	50.8
152	69.1	41.5	6.2	35.2	220	100.0	60.0	9.0	51.0
153	69.5	41.7	6.3	35.5	>220	100.0	60.0	9.0	51.0
154	70.0	42.0	6.3	35.7					
155	70.5	42.3	6.3	35.9					

0.9 mg/kg tPA Dosing Chart

(total IV dose = 0.9 mg/kg, 10% of dose given as bolus, 90% as infusion. Maximum dose is 90 mg)

Wt (lb)	Wt (kg)	Total IV dose	10% Bolus	90% Infusion	Wt (lb)	Wt (kg)	Total IV dose	10% Bolus	90% Infusion
88	40.0	36.0	3.6	32.4	156	70.9	63.8	6.4	57.4
89	40.5	36.4	3.6	32.8	157	71.4	64.2	6.4	57.8
90	40.9	36.8	3.7	33.1	158	71.8	64.6	6.5	58.2
91	41.4	37.2	3.7	33.5	159	72.3	65.0	6.5	58.5
92	41.8	37.6	3.8	33.9	160	72.7	65.5	6.5	58.9
93	42.3	38.0	3.8	34.2	161	73.2	65.9	6.6	59.3
94	42.7	38.5	3.8	34.6	162	73.6	66.3	6.6	59.6
95	43.2	38.9	3.9	35.0	163	74.1	66.7	6.7	60.0
96	43.6	39.3	3.9	35.3	164	74.5	67.1	6.7	60.4
97	44.1	39.7	4.0	35.7	165	75.0	67.5	6.8	60.8
98	44.5	40.1	4.0	36.1	166	75.5	67.9	6.8	61.1
99	45.0	40.5	4.1	36.5	167	75.9	68.3	6.8	61.5
100	45.5	40.9	4.1	36.8	168	76.4	68.7	6.9	61.9
101	45.9	41.3	4.1	37.2	169	76.8	69.1	6.9	62.2
102	46.4	41.7	4.2	37.6	170	77.3	69.5	7.0	62.6
103	46.8	42.1	4.2	37.9	171	77.7	70.0	7.0	63.0
104	47.3	42.5	4.3	38.3	172	78.2	70.4	7.0	63.3
105	47.7	43.0	4.3	38.7	173	78.6	70.8	7.1	63.7
106	48.2	43.4	4.3	39.0	174	79.1	71.2	7.1	64.1
107	48.6	43.8	4.4	39.4	175	79.5	71.6	7.2	64.4
108	49.1	44.2	4.4	39.8	176	80.0	72.0	7.2	64.8
109	49.5	44.6	4.5	40.1	177	80.5	72.4	7.2	65.2
110	50.0	45.0	4.5	40.5	178	80.9	72.8	7.3	65.5
111	50.5	45.4	4.5	40.9	179	81.4	73.2	7.3	65.9
112	50.9	45.8	4.6	41.2	180	81.8	73.6	7.4	66.3
113	51.4	46.2	4.6	41.6	181	82.3	74.0	7.4	66.6
114	51.8	46.6	4.7	42.0	182	82.7	74.5	7.4	67.0
115	52.3	47.0	4.7	42.3	183	83.2	74.9	7.5	67.4
116	52.7	47.5	4.7	42.7	184	83.6	75.3	7.5	67.7
117	53.2	47.9	4.8	43.1	185	84.1	75.7	7.6	68.1
118	53.6	48.3	4.8	43.4	186	84.5	76.1	7.6	68.5
119	54.1	48.7	4.9	43.8	187	85.0	76.5	7.7	68.9
120	54.5	49.1	4.9	44.2	188	85.5	76.9	7.7	69.2
121	55.0	49.5	5.0	44.6	189	85.9	77.3	7.7	69.6
122	55.5	49.9	5.0	44.9	190	86.4	77.7	7.8	70.0
123	55.9	50.3	5.0	45.3	191	86.8	78.1	7.8	70.3
124	56.4	50.7	5.1	45.7	192	87.3	78.5	7.9	70.7
125	56.8	51.1	5.1	46.0	193	87.7	79.0	7.9	71.1
126	57.3	51.5	5.2	46.4	194	88.2	79.4	7.9	71.4
127	57.7	52.0	5.2	46.8	195	88.6	79.8	8.0	71.8
128	58.2	52.4	5.2	47.1	196	89.1	80.2	8.0	72.2
129	58.6	52.8	5.3	47.5	197	89.5	80.6	8.1	72.5
130	59.1	53.2	5.3	47.9	198	90.0	81.0	8.1	72.9
131	59.5	53.6	5.4	48.2	199	90.5	81.4	8.1	73.3
132	60.0	54.0	5.4	48.6	200	90.9	81.8	8.2	73.6
133	60.5	54.4	5.4	49.0	201	91.4	82.2	8.2	74.0
134	60.9	54.8	5.5	49.3	202	91.8	82.6	8.3	74.4
135	61.4	55.2	5.5	49.7	203	92.3	83.0	8.3	74.7
136	61.8	55.6	5.6	50.1	204	92.7	83.5	8.3	75.1
137	62.3	56.0	5.6	50.4	205	93.2	83.9	8.4	75.5
138	62.7	56.5	5.6	50.8	206	93.6	84.3	8.4	75.8
139	63.2	56.9	5.7	51.2	207	94.1	84.7	8.5	76.2
140	63.6	57.3	5.7	51.5	208	94.5	85.1	8.5	76.6
141	64.1	57.7	5.8	51.9	209	95.0	85.5	8.6	77.0
142	64.5	58.1	5.8	52.3	210	95.5	85.9	8.6	77.3
143	65.0	58.5	5.9	52.7	211	95.9	86.3	8.6	77.7
144	65.5	58.9	5.9	53.0	212	96.4	86.7	8.7	78.1
145	65.9	59.3	5.9	53.4	213	96.8	87.1	8.7	78.4
146	66.4	59.7	6.0	53.8	214	97.3	87.5	8.8	78.8
147	66.8	60.1	6.0	54.1	215	97.7	88.0	8.8	79.2
148	67.3	60.5	6.1	54.5	216	98.2	88.4	8.8	79.5
149	67.7	61.0	6.1	54.9	217	98.6	88.8	8.9	79.9
150	68.2	61.4	6.1	55.2	218	99.1	89.2	8.9	80.3
151	68.6	61.8	6.2	55.6	219	99.5	89.6	9.0	80.6
152	69.1	62.2	6.2	56.0	220	100.0	90.0	9.0	81.0
153	69.5	62.6	6.3	56.3	>220	100.0	90.0	9.0	81.0
154	70.0	63.0	6.3	56.7					
155	70.5	63.4	6.3	57.1					

PROCEDURE FOR PREPARING tPA(alteplase) for Ischemic Stroke
Materials list: ALTEPLASE (tPA) Tackle box
2 boxes of 50 mg alteplase-tPA (Activase) contains 50 mg drug and 50 ml diluent (water)
2 dispensing pins
3 luer lock 60 ml syringes
1 syringe 10 ml for bolus
18 gauge syringes
1 empty 100 ml IV bag
alcohol wipes
preprinted labels for bolus dose and infusion dose
Dosing tables for both 0.6 mg/kg and 0.9 mg/kg protocols
STEPS FOR MIXING:
1. Verify patient name and weight and stroke protocol with stroke neurologist.
PROTOCOLS: 0.6 mg/kg, MAX. TOTAL DOSE = 60 mg (15% IV bolus, 85% IV infusion over 30 min)
        OR 0.9 mg/kg , MAX. TOTAL DOSE = 90mg (10% IV bolus, 90% IV infusion over 60 min)

        **if neurologist indicates it is a STROKE STUDY (i.e. IMS II), THIS COMES FROM PHARMACY and neurologist should contact pharmacy directly (ext 22107).

2. Get drug from Pyxis-Access under ALTEPLASE (tPA) 50 mg. The screen will say that you are taking two vials – this equals one ALTEPLASE TACKLE BOX – go ahead and enter that you are taking two vials – if you only use one, it should be returned for credit later (see details later). The door will open and you will see the tackle box labeled ALTEPLASE (tPA) box. It contains everything you need for mixing and preparing the doses only (including written info on calculating dosing).
3. Using enclosed dosing sheet (or calculating doses using appropriate protocol – see reverse side for details), choose appropriate protocol (0.6 mg/kg or 0.9 mg/kg). Locate weight of patient-read across for total dose (note wt. is in lbs 1st column, kg 2nd column). This will tell you how many vials you will have to reconstitute (50 mg or less = 1 vial, >50 mg = 2 vials).
4. Take the vial(s) – there will be two doses (boxes) of alteplase (tPA) in the tackle box (each box with one vial of alteplase powder (tPA) 50 mg and one vial of sterile water (diluent) 50 ml). Locate dispensing pin, remove plastic cover from spike and spike water vial. Unscrew cap from dispensing pin, take luer lock 60 ml syringe and screw into top. Withdraw 50 ml water from vial. Remove syringe and dispensing pin as unit and spike alteplase (tPA) vial. Allow water to flow into vial or gently push water into powder vial (don't push too hard – it will bubble too much). Repeat if second vial needed. Do not discard dispensing pin!
    ****DO NOT SHAKE TO HURRY DISSOLVING – IT WILL INCREASE BUBBLING**
        SWIRL GENTLY TO AVOID BUBBLES
5. While alteplase (tPA) is dissolving, grab the protocol sheet, find the doses you need to draw up, locate the bolus label and IV infusion label. Write patient name and doses on each label.
6. Make sure alteplase (tPA) is dissolved (clear, minimal foam, bubbles). Take labeled 10 ml syringe and withdraw IV bolus dose from vial.
7. Locate empty IV bag, label with IV infusion label. With 60 ml syringe, withdraw dose from vial(s) and inject into empty IV bag using 18 gauge needle.
8. ****Verify IV bolus dose, IV infusion dose, and alteplase (tPA) to be discarded (waste) with another RN prior to infusion.
9. IF ONLY ONE VIAL OF ALTEPLASE (tPA) USED ON PATIENT, RETURN SECOND VIAL TO PYXIS SO PATIENT GETS CREDIT. LEAVE USED BOX ON TOP OF PYXIS SO PHARMACY PERSONNEL CAN FIND TO TAKE BACK AND REFILL. NOTIFY PHARMACY THAT ALTEPLASE BOX NEEDS REFILLING, BY PHONE, FAX OR TUBE.
10. ******NOTIFY PHARMACY IF YOU NOTICE ALTEPLASE (tPA) BOX DOES NOT HAVE LOCKS!!!!!!! IF IT IS NOT LOCKED, IT SHOULD BE REPLACED BY PHARMACY!!
11. IF ALTEPLASE IS NOT USED FOR SOME REASON, PLEASE RETURN TO PHARMACY AFTER CREDITING PATIENT. WE NEED VIAL TO GET CREDIT FROM DRUG COMPANY. ANY QUESTIONS CALL PHARMACY EXT. 22107

CLINICAL ASSESSMENT AND STROKE
SEVERITY SCALES

The Glasgow Coma Scale is useful for some patients with subarachnoid hemorrhage, large intracerebral hemorrhage, and a minority of ischemic strokes.

GLASGOW COMA SCALE

Patient Name: _____

Rater Name: _____

Date: _____

Activity		Score

EYE OPENING

None	1 = Even to supra-orbital pressure	
To pain	2 = Pain from sternum/limb/supra-orbital pressure	
To speech	3 = Non-specific response, not necessarily to command	
Spontaneous	4 = Eyes open, not necessarily aware	_____

MOTOR RESPONSE

None	1 = To any pain; limbs remain flaccid	
Extension	2 = Shoulder adducted and shoulder and forearm internally rotated	
Flexor response	3 = Withdrawal response or assumption of hemiplegic posture	
Withdrawal	4 = Arm withdraws to pain, shoulder abducts	
Localizes pain	5 = Arm attempts to remove supra-orbital/chest pressure	
Obeys commands	6 = Follows simple commands	_____

VERBAL RESPONSE

None	1 = No verbalization of any type	
Incomprehensible	2 = Moans/groans, no speech	
Inappropriate	3 = Intelligible, no sustained sentences	
Confused	4 = Converses but confused, disoriented	
Oriented	5 = Converses and oriented	_____

TOTAL (3–15): _____

REFERENCE

Teasdale G, Jennett B. Assessment of coma and impaired consciousness. A practical scale. The Lancet 1974; 2: 81–4.

Provided by the Internet Stroke Center – www.strokecenter.org

The NIH Stroke Scale (NIHSS) has become a widely accepted tool for assessing stroke severity. It can be easily completed by nurses and/or physicians in 5–10 minutes. On-line training is available from the American Stroke Association (asa.trainingcampus.net) and through NIH (ninds.nih.gov/doctors/stroke_scale_training.htm). As discussed in Chapter 2, all the nurses in the ED, intensive care units (ICUs), and Stroke Center are certified to use the NIHSS at Saint Luke's Hospital. The NIHSS is routinely done on admission to the ED, before and after any intervention, at 24 hours, and at discharge. More frequent assessments can be done if the patient's clinical condition is unstable. Two versions are included here. The first includes the detailed instructions and the second is a more streamlined version that can be used after the clinicians are familiar with the use of the scale.

Mid America Brain and Stroke Institute
NIH STROKE SCALE WORKSHEET
Obtained from Web Site: www.strokecenter.org

Administer stroke scale items in the order listed. Record performance in each category after each subscale exam. Follow directions provided for each exam technique. Scores should reflect what the patient does, not what the clinician thinks the patient can do. Except where indicated, the patient should not be coached (i.e., repeated requests to patient to make a special effort).

Instructions	Scale Definition	Admission Score	24 Hour Score	Discharge Score
1a. Level of Consciousness: The investigator must choose a response, even if a full evaluation is prevented by such obstacles as an endotracheal tube, language barrier, orotracheal trauma/bandages. A 3 is scored only if the patient makes no movement (other than reflexive posturing) in response to noxious stimulation.	0 = **Alert;** keenly responsive. 1 = **Not alert**; but arousable by minor stimulation to obey, answer, or respond. 2 = **Not alert**; requires repeated stimulation to attend, or is obtunded and requires strong or painful stimulation to make movements (not stereotyped). 3 = Responds only with reflex motor or autonomic effects or totally unresponsive, flaccid, and flexic.	___	___	___
1b. LOC Questions: The patient is asked the month and his/her age. The answer must be correct – there is no partial credit for being close. Aphasic and stuporous patients who do not comprehend the questions will score 2. Patients unable to speak because of any cause, language barrier or any other problem not secondary to aphasia are given a 1. It is important that only the initial answer be graded and the examiner not "help" the patient with verbal or non-verbal cues.	0 = **Answers** both questions correctly. 1 = **Answers** one question correctly. 2 = **Answers** neither question correctly.	___	___	___
1c. LOC Commands: The patient is asked to open and close the eyes and then to grip and release the non-paretic hand. Substitute another one step command if the hands cannot be used. Credit is given if an unequivocal attempt is made but not completed due to weakness. If the patient does not respond to command, the task should be demonstrated to them (pantomine) and score the result (i.e., follows none, one or two commands). Patients with trauma, amputation, or other physical impediments should be given suitable one-step commands. Only the first attempt is scored.	0 = **Performs** both tasks correctly. 1 = **Performs** one task correctly. 2 = **Performs** neither task correctly.	___ ___ ___ ___	___	___
2. Best Gaze: Only horizontal eye movements will be tested. Voluntary or reflexive (oculocephalic) eye movement will be scored but caloric testing is not done. If the patient has a conjugate deviation of the eyes that can be overcome by voluntary or reflexive activity, the score will be 1. If a patient has an isolated peripheral nerve paresis (CN III, IV or VI) score a 1. Gaze is testable in all aphasic patients. Patients with ocular trauma, bandages, pre-existing blindness or other disorder of visual acuity or fields should be tested with reflexive movements and a choice made by the investigator. Establishing eye contact and then moving about the patient from side to side will occasionally clarify the presence of a partial gaze palsy.	0 = **Normal.** 1 = **Partial gaze palsy;** gaze is abnormal in one or both eyes, but forced deviation or total gaze paresis is not present. 2 = **Forced deviation,** or total gaze paresis not overcome by the oculocephalic maneuver.	___	___	___

Patient Label

Page 2 of 8		Admission Score	24 Hour Score	Discharge Score
3. Visual: Visual field (upper & lower quadrants) are tested by confrontation, using finger counting or visual threat is appropriate. Patient must be encouraged, but if they look at the side of the moving fingers appropriately, this can be scored as normal. If there is unilateral blindness or enucleation, visual fields in the remaining eye are scored. Score 1 only if a clear-cut asymmetry, including quadrantanopia is found. If patient is blind from any cause score 3. Double simultaneous stimulation is performed at this point. If there is extinction patient receives a 1 and the results are used to answer question 11.	0 = **No visual loss.** 1 = **Partial hemianopia.** 2 = **Complete hemianopia.** 3 = **Bilateral hemianopia (blind including cortical blindness).**	___	___	___
4. Facial Palsy: Ask, or use pantomine to encourage the patient to show teeth or raise eyebrows and close eyes: Score symmetry of grimace in response to noxious stimuli in the poorly responsive or non-comprehending patient. If facial trauma/bandages, orotracheal tube, tape or other physical barrier obscures the face, these should be removed to the extent possible.	0 = **Normal** symmetrical movements. 1 = **Minor paralysis** (flattened nasolabial fold, asymmetry on smiling). 2 = **Partial paralysis** (total or near-total paralysis of lower face). 3 = **Complete paralysis** of one or both sides (absence of facial movement in the upper and lower face).	___	___	___
5. Motor Arm: The limb is placed in the appropriate position: extend the arms (palms down) 90 degrees (if sitting) or 45 degrees (if supine). Drift is scored if the arm falls before 10 seconds. The aphasic patient is encouraged using urgency in the voice and pantomime, but not noxious stimulation. Each limb is tested in turn, beginning with the non-paretic arm. Only in the case of amputation or joint fusion at the shoulder, the examiner should record the score as untestable (UN), and clearly write the explanation for this choice.	0 = **No drift**; limb holds 90 (or 45) degrees for full 10 seconds. 1 = **Drift**; limb holds 90 (or 45) degrees, but drifts down before full 10 seconds; does not hit bed or other support. 2 = **Some effort against gravity**; limb cannot get to or maintain (if cued) 90 (or 45) degrees, drifts down to bed, but has some effort against gravity. 3 = **No effort against gravity**; limb falls. 4 = **No movement.** UN = Amputation or joint fusion, explain: _____ __ **5a. Left Arm** **5b. Right Arm**	___ ___	___ ___	___ ___
6. Motor Leg: The limb is placed in the appropriate position: hold the leg at 30 degrees (always tested supine). Drift is scored if the leg falls before 5 seconds. The aphasic patient is encouraged using urgency in the voice and pantomime, but not noxious stimulation. Each limb is tested in turn, beginning with the non-paretic leg. Only in the case of amputation or joint fusion at the hip, the examiner should record the score as untestable (UN), and clearly write the explanation for this choice.	0 = **No drift**; leg holds 30-degree position for full 5 seconds. 1 = **Drift**; leg falls by the end of the 5-second period but does not hit bed. 2 = **Some effort against gravity**; leg falls to bed by 5 seconds, but has some effort against gravity. 3 = **No effort against gravity**; leg falls to bed immediately. 4 = **No movement.** UN = **Amputation** or joint fusion, explain: _____ __ **6a. Left Leg** **6b. Right Leg**	___ ___	___ ___	___ ___

Patient Label

Page 3 of 8		Admission Score	24 Hour Score	Discharge Score
7. Limb Ataxia: This item is aimed at finding evidence of a unilateral cerebellar lesion. Test with eyes open. In case of visual defect, ensure testing is done in intact visual field. The finger-nose-finger and heel-shin tests are performed on both sides, and ataxia is scored only if present out of proportion to weakness. Ataxia is absent in the patient who cannot understand or is paralyzed. Only in the case of amputation or joint fusion, the examiner should record the score as untestable (UN), and clearly write the explanation for this choice. In case of blindness, test by having the patient touch nose from extended arm position.	0 = **Absent**. 1 = **Present in one limb**. 2 = **Present in two limbs**. UN = **Amputation** or joint fusion, explain: _____			
8. Sensory: Sensation or grimace to pin prick when tested, or withdrawal from noxious stimulus in the obtunded or aphasic patient. Only sensory loss attributed to stroke is scored as abnormal and the examiner should test as many body areas (arms (not hands), legs, trunk, face) as needed to accurately check for hemisensory loss. A score of 2, 'severe or total' should only be given when a severe or total loss of sensation can be clearly demonstrated. Stuporous and aphasic patients will therefore probably score 1 or 0. The patient with brain stem stroke who has bilateral loss of sensation is scored 2. If the patient does not respond and is quadriplegic score 2. Patients in coma (item 1a = 3) are arbitrarily given a 2 on this item.	0 = **Normal**; no sensory loss. 1 = **Mild-to-moderate sensory loss**; patient feels pinprick is less sharp or is dull on the affected side; or there is a loss of superficial pain with pinprick, but patient is aware of being touched. 2 = **Severe to total sensory loss**; patient is not aware of being touched in the face, arm, and leg.			
9. Best Language: A great deal of information about comprehension will be obtained during the preceding sections of the examination. The patient is asked to describe what is happening in the attached picture, to name the items on the attached naming sheet, and to read from the attached list of sentences. Comprehension is judged from responses here as well as to all of the commands in the preceding general neurological exam. If visual loss interferes with the tests, ask the patient to identify objects placed in the hand, repeat, and produce speech. The intubated patient should be asked to write. The patient in coma (question 1a = 3) will arbitrarily score 3 on this item. The examiner must choose a score in the patient with stupor or limited cooperation but a score of 3 should be used only if the patient is mute and follows no one step commands.	0 = **No aphasia, normal** 1 = **Mild to moderate aphasia**; some obvious loss of fluency or facility of comprehension, without significant limitation on ideas expressed or form of expressions. Reduction of speech and/or comprehension, however, makes conversation about provided material difficult or impossible. For example in conversation about provided materials examiner can identify picture or naming card from patient's response. 2 = **Severe aphasia**; all communication is through fragmentary expression; great need for inference, questioning, and guessing by the listener. Range of information that can be exchanged is limited; listener carries burden of communication. Examiner cannot identify materials provided from patient response. 3 = **Mute, global aphasia**; no usable speech or auditory comprehension.			

Patient Label

THE STROKE CENTER HANDBOOK

Page 4 of 8		Admission Score	24 Hour Score	Discharge score
10. Dysarthria: If patient is thought to be normal, an adequate sample of speech must be obtained by asking patient to read or repeat words from the attached list. If the patient has severe aphasia, the clarity of articulation of spontaneous speech can be rated. Only if the patient is intubated or has other physical barriers to producing speech, the examiner should record the score as untestable (UN), and clearly write an explanation for this choice. Do not tell the patient why he or she is being tested.	0 = **Normal.** 1 = **Mild-to-moderate** dysarthria; patient slurs at least some words and, at worst, can be understood with some difficulty. 2 = **Severe dysarthria;** patient's speech is so slurred as to be unintelligible in the absence of or out of proportion to any dysphasia, or is mute/anarthric. UN = **Intubated** or other physical barrier, explain:_____	___	___	___
11. Extinction and inattention (formerly Neglect): Sufficient information to identify neglect may be obtained during the prior testing. If the patient has a severe visual loss preventing visual double simultaneous stimulation, and the cutaneous stimuli are normal, the score is normal. If the patient has aphasia but does appear to attend to both sides, the score is normal. The presence of visual spatial neglect or anosagnosia may also be taken as evidence of abnormality. Since the abnormality is scored only if present, the item is never untestable.	0 =**No Neglect.** 1 = **Visual, tactile, auditory, spatial, or personal inattention** or extinction to bilateral simultaneous stimulation in one of the sensory modalities. 2 = **Profound hemi-inattention or hemi-inattention to more than one modality.** Does not recognize own hand or orients to only one side of space.	___	___	___
TOTAL NIHSS SCORE		___	___	___

Admitting RN Signature Administering Scale _____

24 Hour RN Signature Administering Scale _____

Discharging RN Signature Administering Scale _____

Patient Label

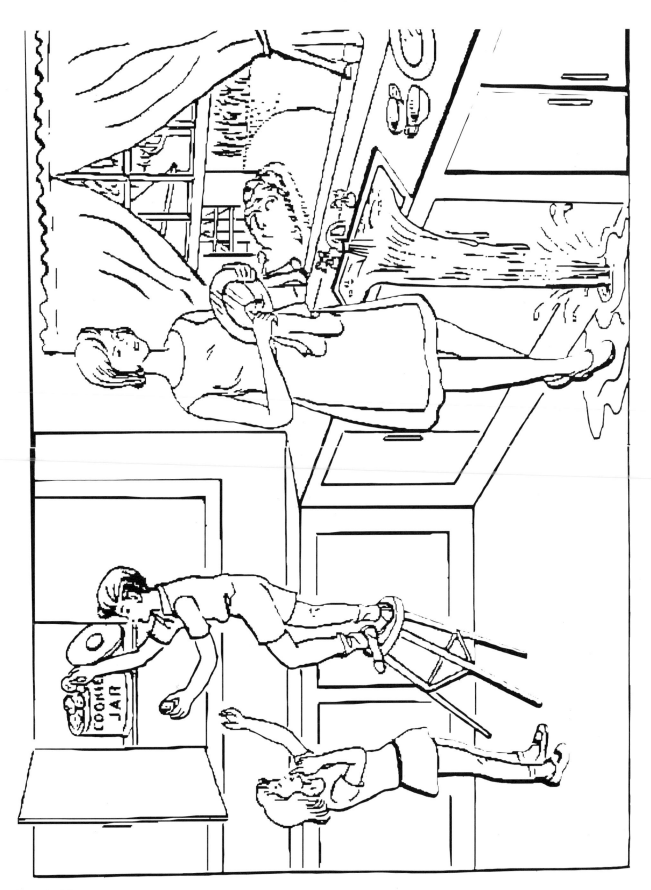

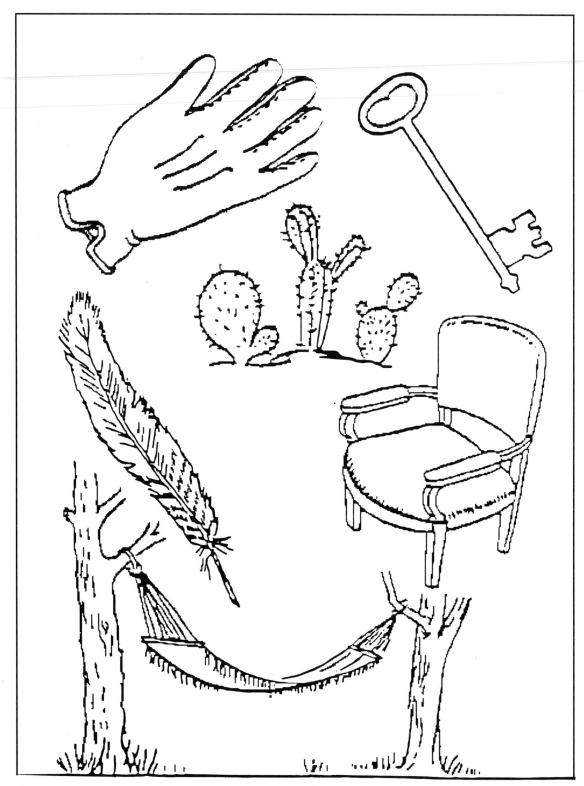

Page 6 of 8

You know how.

Down to earth.

I got home from work.

Near the table in the dining room.

They heard him speak on the radio last
    night.

Page 7 of 8

MAMA

TIP – TOP

FIFTY – FIFTY

THANKS

HUCKLEBERRY

BASEBALL PLAYER

Page 8 of 8

Saint Luke's Hospital
Kansas City, MO 64111

NIH Stroke Scale

CATEGORY	Scale Definition		Admit Score	24 Hour Score	Discharge Score
1a. Level of Consciousness (Alert, drowsy, etc...)	0= Alert 1= Drowsy	2= Stuporous 3= Coma			
1b. LOC Questions (Month, age)	0= Answers both correctly 1= Answers one correctly	2= Answers neither correctly			
1c. LOC Commands (Open close, eyes, make fist, let go)	0= Performs both correctly 1= Performs one correctly	2= Performs neither task correctly			
2. Best Gaze (Eyes open – patient follows examiner's fingers/face)	0= Normal 1= Partial gaze palsy	2= Forced deviation			
3. Visual (Introduce visual stimulus (or threat) to patient's visual field quadrants)	0= No visual loss 1= Partial hemianopia	2= Complete hemianopia 3= Bilateral hemianopia (blind)			
4. Facial Palsy (Show teeth, raise eyebrows, and squeeze eyes shut)	0= Normal 1= Minor paralysis	2= Partial paralysis 3= Complete paralysis			
5. Motor Arm **5a. Left Arm** (Elevate extremity to 90° and score drift/movement)	0= No drift 1= Drift 2= Some effort against gravity	3= No effort against gravity 4= No movement UN= Amputation or joint fusion			
5b. Right Arm (Elevate extremity to 90° and score drift/movement)	0= No drift 1= Drift 2= Some effort against gravity	3= No effort against gravity 4= No movement UN= Amputation or joint fusion			
6. Motor Leg **6a. Left Leg** (Elevate extremity to 30° and score drift/movement)	0= No drift 1= Drift 2= Some effort against gravity	3= No effort against gravity 4= No movement UN= Amputation or joint fusion			
6b. Right Leg (Elevate extremity to 30° and score drift/movement)	0= No drift 1= Drift 2= Some effort against gravity	3= No effort against gravity 4= No movement UN= Amputation or joint fusion			
7. Limb Ataxia (Finger, nose, heel down shin)	0= Absent 1= Present in one limb	2= Present in two limbs UN= Amputation or joint fusion			
8. Sensory (Pinprick to face, arm [trunk] and leg – compare side to side)	0= Normal 1= Mild-to-moderate sensory loss	2= Severe to total sensory loss			
9. Best Language (Name items, describe a picture and read sentences)	0= No aphasia, normal 1= Mild to moderate aphasia	2= Severe aphasia 3= Mute, global aphasia			
10. Dysarthsia (Evaluate speech clarity by patients repeating listed words)	0= Normal 1= Mild-to-moderate	2= Severe dysarthria UN= Intubated			
11. Extinction and Inattention (Use information from prior testing to identify neglect or double simultaneous stimuli)	0= No neglect 1= Partial neglect	2= Profound neglect			
		NIH SCORE			

Patient Label

The Canadian Stroke Scale (CSS) and the Scandinavian Stroke Scale (SSS) have been used in many research trials and share some features with the NIHSS.

THE CANADIAN STROKE SCALE (CSS)

Item	Score (in points)	Item	Score (in points)
Level of consciousness		Motor function (scoring if comprehension is impaired)	
Alert	3	**Face**	
Drowsy	1.5	Symmetricl	0.5
		Asymmetrical	0
Orientation		**Arms**	
Oriented	1	Equal	1.5
Disoriented, not applicable	0	Unequal	0
		Legs	
Language		Equal	1.5
Normal	1	Unequal	0
Expressive deficit	0.5		
Receptive deficit	0		
Motor function (scoring if normal comprehension)			
Face			
No facial weakness	0.5		
Facial weakness present	0		
Proximal arm			
No weakness	1.5		
Mild weakness	1		
Significant weakness	0.5		
Paralysis	0		
Distal arm			
No weakness	1.5		
Mild weakness	1		
Significant weakness	0.5		
Paralysis	0		
Proximal leg			
No weakness	1.5		
Mild weakness	1		
Significant weakness	0.5		
Paralysis	0		
Distal leg			
No weakness	0		
Mild weakness	1		
Significant weakness	0.5		
Paralysis	0		

SCANDINAVIAN STROKE SCALE (SSS)

Item	Score (in points)	Item	Score (in points)
Consciousness		**Orientation**	
Fully conscious	6	Correct for time, place and person	6
Somnolent, can be awaked to full consciousness	4	2 of these	4
		1 of these	2
Reacts to verbal command, but is not fully conscious	2	Completely disorientated	0
		Speech	
Eye movement		No aphasia	10
No gaze palsy	4	Limited vocabulary or incoherent speech	6
Gaze palsy present	2		
Conjugate eye deviation	0	More than yes/no, but not longer sentences	3
		Only yes/no or less	0
Arm, motor power*			
Raises arm with normal strength	6	**Facial palsy**	
Raises arm with reduced strength	5	None-dubious	2
Raises arm with flexion in elbow	4	Present	0
Can move, but not against gravity	2		
Paralysis	0	**Gait**	
		Walks 5 m without aids	12
Hand, motor power*		Walks with aids	9
Normal strength	6	Walks with help of another person	6
Reduced strength in full range	4	Sits without support	3
Some movement, fingertips do not reach palm	2	Bedridden/wheelchair	0
Paralysis	0		
Leg, motor power*			
Normal strength	6		
Raises straight leg with reduced strength	5		
Raises leg with flexion of knee	4		
Can move, but not against gravity	2		
Paralysis	0		

*Motor power is assessed only on the affected side

The Saint Luke's Stroke Center also uses a neuro assessment flowsheet when more frequent evaluations are needed.

The Functional Index Measure (FIM) is widely used in stroke rehabilitation. It is copyrighted and cannot be reproduced.

Frequent Assess. Flowsheet

Saint Luke's Hospital
Kansas City, MO 64111

MABSI Neurological Frequent Assessment Flowsheet

DATA	INITIALS															
	DATE															
	TIME															
VITAL SIGNS	TEMP															
	BP															
	PULSE															
	RESP.															
	O_2 SAT															
PROCEDURE CHECK	PEDAL	R														
	PULSES	L														
	EXT. COLOR															
	EXT. TEMP															
	GROIN DRESSING															
NEUROLOGICAL ASSESSMENT	LOC 0-3															
	LOC 0-2 QUESTIONS															
	LOC 0-2 COMMANDS															
	MOTOR:	RA														
	ARMS 0-4	LA														
	MOTOR:	RL														
	LEGS 0-4	LL														
	FACIAL PALSY 0-3															
	VERBAL 0-3															
	VISUAL FIELD *															
	SENSORY 0-2															
GLASGOW COMA SCALE	EYE OPENING 1-4															
	VERBAL 1-5															
	BEST MOTOR 1-6															
	GCS TOTAL															
	RA MOTOR															
	RL MOTOR															
	LA MOTOR															
	LL MOTOR															
	PUPIL SIZE & REACTION	R														
		L														

Pupil Scale

mm 2 3 4 5 6 7 8 9

PATIENT LABEL

PUPIL REACTION	* Code Key on Back			
	Init.	Signature	Init.	Signature
+ Reactive				
- Nonreactive				
± Sluggish				

Saint Luke's Hospital
Kansas City, MO 64111
FREQUENT NEUROLOGICAL ASSESSMENT KEY

LOC (Level of Consciousness)

0 = Fully alert, immediately responsive to verbal stimuli; is able to cooperate completely.

1 = Drowsy; consciousness is slightly impaired; arouses when stimulated verbally or after shaking; responds appropriately.

> *If the patient scores either 2 or 3 in this section of the neuro check, proceed to the Glasgow Coma Scale*

2 = Stuporous; aroused with difficulty, often painful stimuli must be applied; arousal usually incomplete; responds inadequately; reverts to original state when not stimulated.

3 = Comatose; unresponsive to all stimuli or responds with reflex motor or autonomic effects.

LOC QUESTIONS

0 = Patient knows his age and the month (only initial answer is scored).

1 = Patient answers one question correctly.

2 = Patient unable to speak to understand or answers incorrectly to both questions.

LOC COMMANDS

0 = Patient grips hand and closes/opens eyes to command.

1 = Patient does one correctly.

2 = Patient does neither correctly.

MOTOR: ARM (Right & Left)

The patient is examined with arms outstretched at 90° if sitting or at 45° if lying down. Request full effort for 10 seconds. If consciousness or comprehension is abnormal, cue patient by actively lifting arms into position as the request for effort is verbally given.

0 = No drift (Limb holds at 90° if sitting, at 45° if lying down for full 10 seconds).

1 = Drift (Limb holds position, but drifts before 10 seconds; does not touch the bed).

2 = Some effort against gravity (Limb falls to the bed before 10 seconds).

3 = No effort against gravity (Limb falls, no effort against gravity, some voluntary movement observed).

4 = No movement.

U = Untestable due to amputation.

MOTOR: LEG (Right & Left)

While supine, the patient is asked to maintain the leg at 30° for five seconds. If consciousness or comprehension is abnormal, cue patient by actively lifting leg into position while the request for effort is verbally given.

0 = No drift (Leg holds 30° for five seconds).

1 = Drift (Leg falls to intermediate position by the end of five seconds).

2 = Some effort against gravity (Limb falls to the bed before 10 seconds).

3 = No effort against gravity (Leg falls to bed immediately, with no resistance to gravity, some voluntary movement observed).

4 = No movement.

U = Untestable due to amputation.

FACIAL PALSY	VERBAL	VISUAL FIELD	SENSORY
Ask the patient to show teeth, raise eyebrows, squeeze and shut eyes.	0 = No Aphasia	LFC = Left Field Cut	0 = Normal
	1 = Mild to Moderate	RFC = Right Field Cut	1 = Partial Loss
0 = Normal	2 = Aphasia	B = Blind	2 = Severe Loss
1 = Minor – flattened nasolabial fold	3 = Global Aphasia (Mute)		
2 = Partial – lower face paralysis	D = Dysarthric		
3 = Complete – upper and lower face paralysis			

GLASGOW COMA SCALE		
EYE OPENING	**VERBAL RESPONSE**	**BEST MOTOR RESPONSE**
4 = Spontaneous	5 = Oriented	6 = Obeys
3 = To Speech	4 = Confused Conversation	5 = Localized
2 = To Pain	3 = Inappropriate Words	4 = Withdraw
1 = None	2 = Incomprehensible Sounds	3 = Abnormal Flexion
	1 = None	2 = Abnormal Extension
		1 = None

CODE KEY	SKIN TEMPERATURE
√ Within Normal Limits	W = Warm
* See Nursing Process Notes	C = Cool

OUTCOMES

There are many methods to measure stroke outcomes. The NIHSS at 24 hours and at discharge is a good predictor of overall clinical outcome. Most clinical trials use the Modified Rankin Scale (mRS) and/or the Barthel Index (BI) at 90 days as the standard assessment for clinical outcome. Both of these can be done over the phone if necessary.

MODIFIED RANKIN SCALE (MRS)

Patient Name: _____

Rater Name: _____

Date: _____

Score	Description
0	No symptoms at all
1	No significant disability despite symptoms; able to carry out all usual duties and activities
2	Slight disability; unable to carry out all previous activities, but able to look after own affairs without assistance
3	Moderate disability; requiring some help, but able to walk without assistance
4	Moderately severe disability; unable to walk without assistance and unable to attend to own bodily needs without assistance
5	Severe disability; bedridden, incontinent and requiring constant nursing care and attention
6	Dead

TOTAL (0–6): _____

REFERENCES

Bonita R, Beaglehole R. Modification of Rankin Scale: recovery of motor function after stroke. Stroke 1988; 19: 1497–500.

Rankin J. Cerebral vascular accidents in patients over the age of 60. Scott Med J 1957; 2: 200–15.

Van Swieten JC, Koudstaal PJ, Visser MC, Schouten HJ, van Gijn J. Interobserver agreement for the assessment of handicap in stroke patients. Stroke 1988; 19: 604–7.

Provided by the Internet Stroke Center – www.strokecenter.org

THE BARTHEL INDEX

Patient Name: _____

Rater Name: _____

Date: _____

Activity   Score

FEEDING
   0 = unable
   5 = needs help cutting, spreading butter, etc., or requires modified diet
   10 = independent   _____

BATHING
   0 = dependent
   5 = independent (or in shower)   _____

GROOMING
   0 = needs to help with personal care
   5 = independent face/hair/teeth/shaving (implements provided)   _____

DRESSING
   0 = dependent
   5 = needs help but can do about half unaided
   10 = independent (including buttons, zips, laces, etc.)   _____

BOWELS
   0 = incontinent (or needs to be given enemas)
   5 = occasional accident
   10 = continent   _____

BLADDER
   0 = incontinent, or catheterized and unable to manage alone
   5 = occasional accident
   10 = continent   _____

TOILET USE
   0 = dependent
   5 = needs some help, but can do something alone
   10 = independent (on and off, dressing, wiping)   _____

TRANSFERS (BED TO CHAIR AND BACK)
   0 = unable, no sitting balance
   5 = major help (one or two people, physical), can sit
   10 = minor help (verbal or physical)
   15 = independent   _____

MOBILITY (ON LEVEL SURFACES)
   0 = immobile or < 50 yards
   5 = wheelchair independent, including corners, > 50 yards
   10 = walks with help of one person (verbal or physical) > 50 yards
   15 = independent (but may use any aid; for example, stick) > 50 yards   _____

STAIRS
   0 = unable
   5 = needs help (verbal, physical, carrying aid)
   10 = independent   _____

TOTAL (0–100): _____

Provided by the Internet Stroke Center – www.strokecenter.org

The Barthel ADL Index: Guidelines

1. The index should be used as a record of what a patient does, not as a record of what a patient could do.
2. The main aim is to establish degree of independence from any help, physical or verbal, however minor and for whatever reason.
3. The need for supervision renders the patient not independent.
4. A patient's performance should be established using the best available evidence. Asking the patient, friends/relatives and nurses are the usual sources, but direct observation and common sense are also important. However direct testing is not needed.
5. Usually the patient's performance over the preceding 24-48 hours is important, but occasionally longer periods will be relevant.
6. Middle categories imply that the patient supplies over 50 per cent of the effort.
7. Use of aids to be independent is allowed.

REFERENCES

Collin C, Wade DT, Davies S, Horne V. The Barthel ADL Index: a reliability study. Int Disability Study 1988; 10: 61–3.

Gresham GE, Phillips TF, Labi ML. ADL status in stroke: relative merits of three standard indexes. Arch Phys Med Rehabil 1980; 61: 355–8.

Loewen SC, Anderson BA. Predictors of stroke outcome using objective measurement scales. Stroke 1990; 21: 78–81.

Mahoney FI, Barthel D. Functional evaluation: the Barthel Index. Maryland State Med J 1965; 14: 56–61.

Copyright information

CLINICAL PATHS AND ORDER SETS

At the Saint Luke's Stroke Center the clinical paths are used by the nurses as a charting tool. Each clinical path has an associated order set used by the physicians.

The Stroke Group at the NINDS led by Dr Steve Warach has developed an ischemic stroke pathway that is updated yearly. It is not available on their website. Included here is the clinical path from that document.

Saint Luke's Hospital Kansas City, MO – Clinical Path – Stroke

Inclusion Criteria: Ischemic Stroke and Non-Surgical Hemorrhagic Stroke
Excluded: Surgical Hemorrhagic Stroke

Problem: Disrupted Cerebral Perfusion
Nursing Diagnosis: **Altered Cerebral Tissue Perfusion** related to ischemia or hemorrhage
Initiated Date: _____ Modified: _____ Resolved: _____
Key Outcome Statement: Cerebral perfusion will remain adequate as evidenced by:

Expected Outcome:
1. Neuro function IER-LOC/motor/sensory/visual/cognitive
2. Patient free of signs and symptoms of increased ICP
3. Vital Signs remain in prescribed range
4. Pt will not demonstrate seizure activity

Nursing Assessment/
Intervention
(Practice Interventions)
1. Assess neuro status/function trends – LOC, motor (movement, muscle tone, drift) sensory, pupils size, shape, symmetry, reactivity), cognition every 4 hours
2. Assess VS-BP, HR, respiratory rate and pattern, temp every 4 hours
3. Maintain body alignment in midline and avoid neck flexion or head rotation – ongoing
4. Plan nursing care, procedure for energy conservation to minimize increased ICP every 12 hours
5. Prevent accumulation of tracheobronchial secretions every 4 hours
6. Administer prescribed medications/fluids (volume expanders, vasoactive medication, anticoagulants, sedative, analgesics, etc.) to maintain hemodynamic parameters and optimize cerebral perfusion as ordered

Problem: Communication
Nursing Diagnosis: **Impaired verbal communication** related to neurological impairment
Initiated Date: _____ Modified: _____ Resolved: _____
Key Outcome Statement: Ability to receive, interpret and express messages will improve as evidenced by:

Expected Outcome:
1. Communicates understanding of messages received
2. Use of non-verbal, verbal and written communication

Nursing Assessment/
Intervention
(Practice Interventions)
1. Assess ability to comprehend/communicate daily
2. Speak slowly, using short sentences ongoing
3. Provide communication board once

Problem: Disrupted Peripheral Perfusion
Nursing Diagnosis: **Ineffective peripheral tissue perfusion** related to reduction/interruption of venous/arterial blood flow
Initiated Date: _____ Modified: _____ Resolved: _____
Key Outcome Statement: Peripheral tissue perfusion is adequate to nourish the tissue as evidence by:

Expected Outcome:
1. Peripheral perfusion IER (color/temp/capillary refill/pulses)
2. Skin intact
3. Absence of peripheral edema
4. Absence of localized extremity pain
5. Sensation level IER
6. Motor function IER

Nursing Assessment/
Intervention
(Practice Interventions)
1. Assess peripheral perfusion, i.e. peripheral pulses, color, temperature, capillary refill every 8 hours
2. Inspect skin for tissue breakdown or ulcers every 12 hours
3. Assess pain level q 12h
4. Assess sensation and motor function every 8 hours
5. Maintain TED hose/SCDs
6. Assess for signs of peripheral embolus
7. Implement appropriate wound care; consider need for multidisciplinary consult i.e. skin nurse, pharmacy

Path intermediate/discharge goals reviewed with patient/SO and mutually agreed upon.
Date: _____ **RN Signature:** _____

SAINT LUKE'S HOSPITAL OF KANSAS CITY
Office of Clinical Practice Guidelines

PATIENT LABEL

The suggested plan represents the initial desired course of treatment and goals of recovery. These are representative or average guidelines only and should be reviewed periodically by the attending physician and other involved disciplines. Deviations are generally expected and revisions to the plan should be made as warranted

Saint Luke's Hospital Kansas City, MO - Clinical Path –Stroke

Problem: Inability to swallow effectively

Nursing Diagnosis: **Risk for Aspiration** related to disease process

Initiated Date: _____ Modified: _____ Resolved: _____

Key Outcome Statement: Patient will not aspirate as evidenced by:

Expected Outcome:
1. Lung sounds IER
2. Respiratory rate, rhythm IER
3. Absence of onset of new fever/cough

Nursing Assessment/ Intervention (Practice Interventions)
1. Assess pulmonary status every 8 hours
2. Keep HOB elevated 30 ° at all times continuously
3. Maintain patent airway-ongoing
4. Assess LOC, cough reflex, gag reflex and swallowing ability every 8 hours
5. collaborate with speech therapy to assess swallow ability within 24 hours of admission. Keep patient NPO if demonstrates risk of aspiration-once
6. Position upright 90 degrees or as far as possible for at least 15 minutes before and after feeding with meals
7. Implement oral care protocol once
8. Suction set-up to bedside daily
9. Verify placement of enteral tube prior to feeding/administering meds daily
10. Collaborate with physician for peptic ulcer prophylaxis once

Problem: Inability to eat

Nursing Diagnosis: **Imbalanced nutrition, less than body requirements** related to disease process

Initiated Date: _____ Modified: _____ Resolved: _____

Key Outcome Statement: Nutrient intake meets metabolic needs as evidenced by:

Expected Outcome:
1. Pt/SO/Family/ caregiver expresses understanding of nutritional deficit/plan
2. Fluid and food intake IER
3. Blood glucose IER
4. Pt/SO/caregiver demonstrates ability to maintain adequate nutritional intake

Nursing Assessment/ Intervention (Practice Interventions)
1. Record percent of meal eaten TID
2. Assess weight as ordered but at least weekly
3. Collaborate with dietitian on nutritional assessment, counseling and/or plan once
4. Assess blood glucose per orders and PRN
5. Assess abdomen, bowel sounds, and bowel elimination q 12 hours

Problem: Decreased mobility

Nursing Diagnosis: **Impaired physical mobility** related to disease process

Initiated Date: _____ Modified: _____ Resolved: _____

Key Outcome Statement: Mobility is maintained or increased as evidenced by:

Expected Outcome:
1. Pt will demonstrate balance/strength development and ambulation activities IER
2. No evidence of complications from impaired mobility
3. Participates in establishing activity goals
4. Pt/SO verbalizes and demonstrates understanding of safety measures and physical limitations

Nursing Assessment/ Intervention (Practice Interventions)
1. Assess and record amount of daily activity
2. Teach Pt/SO sign/symptoms of complications from impaired mobility daily
3. Collaborate with PT/OT and rehab to assess progress with mobility daily
4. Assess for complications of immobility every 12 hours
5. Collaborate with PT and patient to assess and set goals related to balance, strength and mobility daily
6. Assess for complications of immobility
7. Complete risk assessment and collaborate with physician for DVT prophylaxis

Problem: Decreased knowledge

Nursing Diagnosis: **Knowledge Deficit** related to lack of information/no knowledge of resources

Initiated Date: _____ Modified: _____ Resolved: _____

Key Outcome Statement: Pt/SO demonstrates knowledge and or skills needed to practice heath behaviors as evidenced by:

Expected Outcome:
1. Pt/SO verbalized understanding of procedures and disease process
2. Pt/SO verbalizes/demonstrates ability to care for self/pt
3. Pt/SO sets realistic goals

Nursing Assessment/ Intervention (Practice Interventions)
1. Assess pt/so current knowledge level daily
2. Provide individualized instruction on specific aspect of care daily
3. Review, reinforce and modify teaching methods as needed daily
4. Assess readiness and ability to learn daily
5. Collaborate with PT/SO to develop realistic learning objectives daily
6. Evaluate Pt/SO ability to verbalize/demonstrate understanding of information/instruction taught-once

Patient Label

Saint Luke's Hospital Kansas City, MO – Clinical Path – Stroke

	NURSING DIAGNOSIS/ OUTCOME STATEMENT	Intensive-Close Monitoring Phase DATE: _____ to _____ W1 W2	Explain unmet EOs
NEURO/COGNITIVE PITCH	**Nursing Diagnosis: Ineffective cerebral tissue perfusion** related to ischemia or hemorrhage	**Intervention:** [ ] Request to initiate Stroke Standing Orders if not done in ED [ ] [ ] Neuro assess q 1 hr x 8 then q 2 **(ICU)** [ ] [ ] Neuro assess q 2 hour x 4 then q 4 **(M/S)** [ ] [ ] Adm. NIH Stroke Score _____ [ ] CT ordered or if done initial results to chart	_____ _____ _____ _____ _____
	Outcome Statement: Cerebral perfusion will be adequate as evidenced by:	**Expected Outcomes:** ___ ___ **No deterioration in neuro assessment** ___ ___ **Patient free of signs/symptoms of increased ICP** ___ ___ **VS in prescribed range** ___ ___ **Pt free from seizure activity**	_____ _____ _____ _____
	Nursing Diagnosis: Impaired Verbal Communication related to disease process	**Intervention:** [ ] [ ] Speak slow, use short sentences/allow extra time to respond [ ] Communication Disorders consult and treat [ ] [ ] Demonstrate to Pt/SO use of communication tools/ techniques	_____ _____ _____
	Outcome Statement: Ability to receive, interpret and express information will improve as evidenced by:	**Expected Outcomes:** ___ ___ Communicates understanding of information received ___ ___ Use of verbal and nonverbal communication	_____ _____
CARDIO/ PULMONARY	**Nursing Diagnosis: Ineffective peripheral tissue perfusion** related to reduction/interruption of blood flow	**Intervention:** [ ] [ ] Vital signs q 15 min. x 4; q 30 min x 2 if stable **(ICU)** [ ] [ ] Vital signs q 2 hour x 4; q 4 hours if stable **(M/S)** [ ] [ ] Obtain BP range orders from Physician [ ] [ ] Adm O_2 sat _____ and q shift [ ] [ ] DVT precautions, TED's if IV tPA used, SCD's if no IV tPA	_____ _____ _____ _____ _____
	Outcome Statement: Tissue Perfusion will remain adequate as evidenced by:	**Expected Outcomes:** ___ ___ **BP within desired range according to orders** ___ ___ $SPO_2 \geq 92\%$ on $\leq$ 5L NC, wean if > 92% ___ ___ **Cardiac rhythm stable with HR $\geq$ 60 and $\leq$ 120**	_____ _____ _____
GI/GU/NUTRITION	**Nursing Diagnosis: Risk for aspiration** related to disease process	**Intervention:** [ ] [ ] Assess cough and gag reflex q shift and PRN [ ] [ ] Keep NPO if patient demonstrates aspiration risk [ ] [ ] Consult Communication Disorders for bedside swallow eval [ ] Communication Disorders consult entered	_____ _____ _____ _____
	Outcome Statement: Pt. will not aspirate as evidenced by:	**Expected Outcomes:** ___ ___ Lung sounds IER/Moves sputum out of airway ___ ___ SOA not present	_____ _____
	Nursing Diagnosis: Imbalanced nutrition, less than required related to disease process	**Intervention:** [ ] Dietician consult/nutrition plan NPO _____ or Diet _____ [ ] PBG on admission _____ and QID if diabetic [ ] Assess for incontinence, request order for Foley PRN [ ] Last BM _____, give laxative if > 48 hours	_____ _____ _____ _____
	Outcome Statement: Nutrient intake meets needs as evidenced by:	**Expected Outcomes:** ___ ___ Pt/SO expresses understanding of nutritional plan	_____
SKIN/ MUSCULO/ SKELETAL	**Nursing Diagnosis: Impaired Physical Mobility** related to disease	**Intervention:** [ ] PT and OT Consult entered/Rehab MD consult entered	_____
	Outcome Statement: Mobility is maintained or increased as evidenced by:	**Expected Outcomes:** ___ ___ Participates in ADLs ___ ___ No evidence of complications from immobility	_____ _____
TEACHING	**Nursing Diagnosis: Deficient knowledge** related to lack of information	**Intervention:** [ ] Assess Pt/SO knowledge level of disease/diagnostic tests [ ] Provide stroke appropriate educational materials for Pt/SO [ ] Patient Path reviewed with Pt/SO	_____ _____ _____
	Outcome Statement: Pt/SO demonst knowledge/skills needed to practice health behaviors as evidenced by:	**Expected Outcomes:** ___ ___ Pt/SO verb understanding of dx procedures/disease process ___ ___ Pt/SO verb/demon understands of safety measures/limits	Initial Signature _____

SYMBOL KEY: ___ = Expected Outcome [ ] = Interventions	A in a [√] indicates intervention done A "o" in a [ ] or on a line indicates not pertinent	"Initials" on line means Expected Outcome done/findings as expected A "*" in a [ ] or on a line indicates the item not done as expected.

Patient Label

Saint Luke's Hospital Kansas City, MO – Clinical Path – Stroke

	NURSING DIAGNOSIS/ OUTCOME STATEMENT	Diagnostic-Evaluation Phase DATE: ________ to ________ INITIAL W1 W2	Explain unmet EOs Indicate time/nursing dx with key
NEURO/COGNITIVE PSYCH	**Nursing Diagnosis:** **Ineffective cerebral tissue perfusion** related to ischemia or hemorrhage	**Intervention:** [ ] [ ] Neuro assessment q 4 hour if no deterioration [ ] NIH Stroke Scale repeated at 24 hours or prior to DC if earlier (**ICU**) [ ] Follow-up imaging if t-PA [ ] CT head [ ] MRI head [ ] MRA	
	Outcome Statement: Cerebral perfusion will be adequate	**Expected Outcomes:** __ __ **No deterioration in neuro assessment** __ __ **VS in prescribed range** **No seizure activity**	
	Nursing Diagnosis: Impaired Verbal Communication related to disease process	**Intervention:** [ ] [ ] Communication Disorders consult completed [ ] [ ] Communication techniques posted in room [ ] [ ] Reinforce Pt/SO use of communication tools/techniques	
	Outcome Statement: Ability to receive, interpret and express information will improve as evidenced by:	**Expected Outcomes:** __ __ Improved ability to communicate verbally or nonverbally __ __ Communication Disorder eval/reports on chart	
CARDIO/ PULMONARY	**Nursing Diagnosis: Ineffective peripheral tissue perfusion** related to interrupted blood flow	**Intervention:** [ ] [ ] Vital signs q 2 (**ICU**)/q 4 hours (**M/S**) if stable [ ] [ ] Telemetry monitoring [ ] [ ] O_2 sat q shift and PRN [ ] [ ] SCD's placed bilaterally if not up ad lib	
	Outcome Statement: Tissue Perfusion will remain adequate as evidenced by:	**Expected Outcomes:** __ __ **BP within desired range according to orders** __ __ $SPO_2 \geq 92\%$ on $\leq$ 5L NC, wean if > 92% __ __ **Cardiac rhythm stable with HR $\geq$ 60 and $\leq$ 120**	
GI/GU/NUTRITION	**Nursing Diagnosis: Risk for aspiration** related to disease process	**Intervention:** [ ] [ ] Follow Communication Disorders recommendation if at risk for asp. [ ] [ ] Request Dobhoff/NG placement if failed swallowgram [ ] [ ] Assess cough/gag daily/PRN, Suction excess secretions PRN	
	Outcome Statement: Pt. will not aspirate as evidenced by:	**Expected Outcomes:** __ __ Lung sounds IER/SOA not present/Moves sputum out of airway __ __ Swallowgram report on chart __ __ Pt/SO/Family acknowledge risk for aspiration __ __ Resp rate/rhythm/effort IER	
	Nursing Diagnosis: Imbalanced nutrition, less than required related to disease process	**Intervention:** [ ] [ ] Collaborate with Physician/family for long term feeding plan [ ] [ ] Give laxative if no BM > 48 hours [ ] [ ] Discontinue Foley if patient alert/cognitive and mobility allows [ ] [ ] Assess bladder incontinence and retention	
	Outcome Statement: Nutrient intake meets metabolic needs as evidenced by:	**Expected Outcomes:** __ __ **Pt/SO understands nutritional deficit and feeding plan** __ __ Demonstrates normal bowel function __ __ UOP adequate	
SKIN/ MUSCULO/ SKELETAL	**Nursing Diagnosis: Impaired Physical Mobility** related to disease	**Intervention:** [ ] [ ] PT/OT/Rehab MD evaluation completed	
	Outcome Statement: Mobility is maintained or increased as evidenced by:	**Expected Outcomes:** __ __ Participates in ADLs __ __ No evidence of complications from impaired mobility __ __ Tolerates chair or dangle 15 – 30 min BID	
TEACHING	**Nursing Diagnosis: Deficient knowledge** related to lack of information **Outcome Statement:** Pt/SO/Family demonstrates knowledge and/or skills needed to practice health behaviors as evidenced by:	Intervention: [ ] [ ] Discuss with Pt/SO ICU to stroke center transfer concerns [ ] [ ] Assess knowledge of stroke etiology/dx tests; provide educ mat. [ ] [ ] Discuss safety measures/mobility/alternative commun tech [ ] [ ] Consult CM and SW to assist with DC planning Expected Outcomes: __ __ Demonstrates safety measures, verbalizes rehab team plan __ __ PT/SO demonstrates alternative communication tech/resources __ __ Pt/SO verbalizes understanding diag tests/disease process	Initial Signature

Patient Label

Saint Luke's Hospital Kansas City, MO – Clinical Path – Stroke

	NURSING DIAGNOSIS/ OUTCOME STATEMENT	Transitional-Rehabilitation Phase DATE: _____ to _____ W1 W2	Explain unmet EOs
NEURO/COGNITIVE PSYCH	**Nursing Diagnosis: Ineffective cerebral tissue perfusion** related to ischemia or hemorrhage **Outcome Statement:** Cerebral perfusion will be adequate:	Intervention: [ ][ ] Neuro Assessment q 4 hours **record on Neuro Flow sheet** Expected Outcomes: __ __ **No deterioration in neuro assessment** __ __ **Patient free of S/S of increased ICP** __ __ **VS in prescribed range** __ __ **No seizure activity**	
	Nursing Diagnosis: Impaired Verbal Communication related to disease process **Outcome Statement:** Ability to receive/interpret/express info will improve:	Intervention: [ ][ ] Reinforce Pt/SO use of communication tools/techniques [ ][ ] Communication Disorders evaluation on chart Expected Outcomes: __ __ Improved ability to communicate verbally or nonverbally	
CARDIO/ PULMONARY	**Nursing Diagnosis: Ineffective peripheral tissue perfusion** related to interrupted blood flow **Outcome Statement:** Tissue Perfusion will remain adequate as evidenced by:	Intervention: [ ][ ] Telemetry monitoring if IER after 72 hours DC [ ][ ] O$_2$ sat q shift and PRN [ ][ ] SCD's placed bilaterally if not up ad lib Expected Outcomes: __ __ **BP within desired range according to orders** __ __ SPO$_2$ $\geq$ 92% on $\leq$ 5L NC, wean if > 92% __ __ **Cardiac rhythm stable with HR $\geq$ 60 and $\leq$ 120**	
GI/GU/NUTRITION	**Nursing Diagnosis: Risk for aspiration** related to disease process **Outcome Statement:** Pt. will not aspirate as evidenced by:	Intervention: [ ][ ] Keep HOB > 30 degrees, 90 degrees during meals if not NPO [ ][ ] Assess cough/gag daily/PRN, Suction excess secretions PRN Expected Outcomes: __ __ Lung sounds IER/SOA not present __ __ Resp rate rhythm/effort IER __ __ Moves sputum out of airway __ __ Pt/SO/Family acknowledge risk for aspiration	
	Nursing Diagnosis: Imbalanced nutrition, less than required related to disease process **Outcome Statement:** Nutrient intake meets metabolic needs as evidenced by:	Intervention: [ ][ ] Give laxative if no BM > 48 hours [ ][ ] Discontinue Foley if patient alert/cognitive and mobility allows [ ][ ] Assess bladder incontinence and retention Expected Outcomes: __ __ **Eats at least 50% of diet or able to tolerate tube feeding** __ __ Demonstrates normal bowel function __ __ UOP adequate	
SKIN/ MUSCULO/ SKELETAL	**Nursing Diagnosis: Impaired Physical Mobility** related to disease process **Outcome Statement:** Mobility is maintained or increased as evidenced by:	Intervention: [ ][ ] PT/OT evaluation on chart [ ][ ] Collaborate with PT/OT to assess progress with mobility/activity Expected Outcomes: __ __ Participates in ADLs __ __ No evidence of complication from impaired mobility __ __ Demonstrates maintenance/improvement of strength/balance __ __ Demonstrates increasing independence with ADLs/self care __ __ Actively participates in ADLs/therapies in a positive manner __ __ Tolerates chair BID ____ 15 min ____ 30 min ____ 60 min	Initial Signature
TEACHING	**Nursing Diagnosis: Deficient knowledge** related to lack of information **Outcome Statement:** Pt/SO/Family demonstrates knowledge and/or skills needed to practice health behaviors as evidenced by:	Intervention: [ ][ ] Review Pt disease process/test results/educational pamphlets [ ][ ] (RN, CM, SSW, PT, OT, Speech discuss with Pt/SO rehab needs [ ][ ] Reinforce/Teach Pt/SO safety measures relevant to pts mobility [ ][ ] Start Stroke Risk Reduction Plan sheet addressing risk factors Expected Outcomes: __ __ Pt/SO understands relevant safety measures (mobility/nutrition) __ __ Pt/SO/Family actively discuss rehab needs and possible options __ __ Pt/SO verbalize stroke etiology/test results/stroke risk factors	SYMBOL KEY: __ = Expected Outcom [ ] = Interventions A √ in a [ ] indicates intervention done A "o" in a [ ] or line indicates pertinent "Initials" on line = EO as expected A "*" in a [ ] or line = not expected.

Patient Label

Saint Luke's Hospital Kansas City, MO – Clinical Path – Stroke

	NURSING DIAGNOSIS/ OUTCOME STATEMENT	Discharge Phase DATE: _____ to_____ INITIAL W1 W2	Explain unmet EOs
NEURO/COGNITIVE PSYCH	**Nursing Diagnosis: Ineffective cerebral tissue perfusion** related to ischemia or hemorrhage	**Intervention:** [ ][ ] Neuro Assessment q 8 hr **record on Neuro Freq Flow sheet** [ ][ ] Complete NIH Stroke Scale on day of discharge	_____ _____
	Outcome Statement: Cerebral perfusion will be adequate as evidenced by:	**Expected Outcomes:** __ __ **No deterioration in neuro assessment** __ __ **Patient free of S/S of increased ICP** __ __ **VS in prescribed range** __ __ **No seizure activity**	_____ _____ _____ _____
	Nursing Diagnosis: Impaired Verbal Communication r/t disease	**Intervention:** [ ][ ] Reinforce Pt/SO use of communication tools/technique s	_____
	Outcome Statement: Ability to receive/interpret/express info improved	**Expected Outcomes:** __ __ Improved ability to communicate verbally or nonverbally	_____
CARDIO/ PULMONARY	**Nursing Diagnosis: Ineffective peripheral tissue perfusion** related to interrupted blood flow	**Intervention:** [ ][ ] Vital signs q 8 hours/O$_2$ sat q shift and PRN [ ][ ] SCD's placed bilaterally if not up ad lib	_____ _____
	Outcome Statement: Tissue Perfusion will remain adequate as evidenced by:	**Expected Outcomes:** __ __ **BP within desired range according to orders** __ __ **SPO$_2$ $\geq$ 92% on $\leq$ 5L NC, wean if > 92%** __ __ **Cardiac rhythm stable with HR $\geq$ 60 and $\leq$ 120 or IER**	_____ _____ _____
GI/GU/NUTRITION	**Nursing Diagnosis: Risk for aspiration** related to disease process	**Intervention:** [ ][ ] Keep HOB > 30 degrees, 90 degrees during meals if not NPO [ ][ ] Assess cough/gag daily/PRN, Suction excess secretions PRN	_____ _____
	Outcome Statement: Pt. will not aspirate as evidenced by:	**Expected Outcomes:** __ __ Lung sounds IER/SOA not present/Moves sputum out of airway __ __ Pt/SO/Family acknowledge risk for aspiration __ __ Resp rate/rhythm/effort IER	_____ _____ _____
	Nursing Diagnosis: Imbalanced nutrition, less than required related to disease process	**Intervention:** [ ][ ] Give laxative if no BM > 48 hours [ ][ ] Discontinue Foley, if patient alert/cognitive and mobility allows [ ][ ] Assess bladder incontinence and retention	_____ _____ _____
	Outcome Statement: Nutrient intake meets metabolic needs as evidenced by:	**Expected Outcomes:** __ __ **Pt/SO demonstrates ability to maintain nutritional intake** __ __ **Demonstrates normal bowel function** __ __ **UOP adequate**	_____ _____ _____
SKIN/ MUSCULO/ SKELETAL	**Nursing Diagnosis: Impaired Physical Mobility** related to disease process	**Intervention:** [ ][ ] Collaborate with PT/OT to assess progress with mobility/activity	_____
	Outcome Statement: Mobility is maintained or increased as evidenced by:	**Expected Outcomes:** __ __ **No evidence of complication from impaired mobility** __ __ Demonstrates maintenance/improvement of strength/balance __ __ Demonstrates increasing independence with ADLs/self care __ __ Participates in ADLs/therapies in a positive manner __ __ Tolerates chair TID _____15 min _____30 min _____60 min	_____ _____ _____ _____ _____
TEACHING	**Nursing Diagnosis: Deficient knowledge** related to lack of information **Outcome Statement:** Pt/SO/Family demonstrates knowledge and/or skills needed to practice health behaviors as evidenced by:	**Intervention:** [ ][ ] Complete Stroke Risk Reduction Plan sheet/give to pt at DC [ ][ ] Pt/SO/Family agree on rehab plan and patient disposition [ ][ ] Discuss diagnostic evaluations and testing after discharge [ ][ ] Reinforce/Teach Pt/SO discharge safety measures **Expected Outcomes:** __ __ **Pt/SO verbalizes risk factors and plan for life style changes** __ __ **Pt/SO verbalizes and agrees on discharge plan** __ __ **Pt/SO understands safety measures relevant to pts mobility**	Initial Signature _____ _____

Patient Label

Saint Luke's Hospital of Kansas City
SAINT LUKE'S-SHAWNEE MISSION HEALTH SYSTEM

Patient Path for Stroke
Average Hospital Stay Range: 4–5 days

Patient: _____

Saint Luke's Hospital staff and doctors are dedicated to giving you the best possible care. This path is to help you and your family become more involved in your care. Since each person is an individual, your care may differ from this general guideline.

HEALTH TEAM MEMBERS

Registered Nurse (RN):
Your nurses are responsible for your nursing care. They plan and coordinate your care with all health team members as well as with you and your family.

Patient Care Technician (PCT):
PCTs will help you with personalized care and daily needs. They may perform procedures such as blood pressure, temperature, drawing of blood, and EKGs.

Registered Dietitian/Diet Technician:
A dietitian/diet technician works with your doctor to meet your nutritional needs. They will evaluate your nutrition status. They will check the advancement and tolerance of your diet or feeding other than by mouth. They can answer any questions about your nutrition needs.

Case Management Department:
A case manager will work with your physician and your insurance company to facilitate proper filing and documentation of your hospital stay. They can address any questions or concerns regarding your insurance or coverage.

Physical, Occupational, and Speech Therapists:
Will be responsible for checking your mobility and coordination, ability to perform self care tasks, and communication skills. The therapist will plan your therapy and set goals to assist in discharge.

Social Worker:
Social workers provide counseling, information, education, support, and referrals to you and your family as you adjust to the impact of your illness or treatment. The social worker will assist you in making plans for your care after you leave the hospital.

Patient Advocate:
The patient advocate is your personal connection to the hospital system. If you have a question about your hospital stay, please call (816) 932-2328.

Chaplain:
A hospital chaplain is available 24 hours a day to provide spiritual guidance and emotional support for you and your family.

STROKE

CARE CATEGORY	HOSPITAL STAY GOALS	INTENSIVE	INTENSIVE TREATMENT	DIAGNOSTIC/ EVALUATION
ASSESSMENT	Stabilize and monitor symptoms	• Neurological and physical exams • Heart monitor • Blood pressure, heart rate, temperature	• Neuro and physical exams • Heart monitor • Vital signs	• Neuro and physical exams • Vital signs
TESTS/LAB	Determine cause of stroke	• Brain scans • Lab work, blood sugar, oxygen concentration, cholesterol levels • Bedside swallowing test	• Tests to visualize flow of blood in neck, brain, and heart – MRI, MRA, carotid Doppler • May have a swallowing test in radiology	• Tests to visualize the heart – ECHO or transesophageal echo (TEE) • Blood test if on blood thinner
FOOD AND DRINK	Maintain nutritional status	• Will not be able to take any fluid or food to swallowing evaluated by speech therapist • If unable to eat may be fed by a tube placed in the stomach	• Food type based on swallowing exam results • If concerns about swallowing and feeding wishes, talk to nurse and physician	• If concerns about diet ask to talk to dietitian • Follow speech therapy swallowing techniques • Discuss long term feeding plan
ACTIVITY	Move toward self care	• Bedrest • Turned from side to side every 2 hours • Dangle on side of bed	• Physical therapist will begin mobility at bedside • Chair 2 times a day	• Therapy in the rehabilitation department (4th floor) • Chair 3 times a day
STROKE TEAM MEMBERS	Begin rehabilitation process	• Evaluation at bedside by rehab team members (physical, occupational, and speech therapist) • Evaluation by physician specializing in rehab	• Therapist will begin therapy at bedside • Education by team members on actions to make you safe following your stroke	• Social service worker and case manager will begin to plan rehabilitation and discharge needs • Rehabilitation physician will plan rehabilitation therapy
MEDICATION	To reduce risk of further complications and decrease risk of future stroke	• Medication to treat identified cause of stroke (blood thinner, antiplatelets, blood pressure, elevated cholesterol, diabetes management)	• Medication continued to treat stroke risk factors	• Medication continued to treat stroke risk factors
DISCHARGE PLANNING AND LEARNING	Discuss physical needs, home environment, and equipment necessary to return home	• Stroke education brochures • Nurse will discuss plan of care during hospitalization, and safety measures • Inform nurse of normal bowel and bladder habits	• Nurses and therapist will educate on stroke disease and risk factors	• Discuss with nurse/social worker post-hospital care needs or transfer to rehabilitation or skilled nursing unit

The suggested plan represents the initial desired course of treatment and goals of recovery. These are representative of average guidelines only. They should be reviewed periodically by the attending physician and other involved care providers. Deviations are generally expected and revisions to the plan should be made as warranted.

STROKE

CARE CATEGORY	TRANSITIONAL	TRANSITIONAL	PATIENT/FAMILY DISCHARGE GOALS
ASSESSMENT	• Neuro and physical exams • Heart monitor – discontinued if normal heart rhythm	• Neuro and physical exams	• Understands signs and symptoms and own risk factors of stroke
TESTS/LAB	• Blood test if on blood thinner	• Education on blood test needed after discharge	• Understands what follow up lab and next doctor appointment required
FOOD AND DRINK	• Feeding plan should be established		• Understands discharge nutrition plan and swallowing instructions
ACTIVITY	• Chair 3 times a day • Therapy in Rehab Department – education on mobility safety and assistive device equipment	• Education on mobility and safety measures	• Understands mobility techniques and safety measures to take at home • Understands activity and exercise options
STROKE TEAM MEMBERS	• Social Service/Home Health will discuss final discharge/ rehabilitation needs	• Most patients discharged	• Understands further home needs or rehabilitation plan
MEDICATION	• Medications discussed and the reason for education	• Discuss adverse effect of medications and what to monitor	• Understands purpose, medication schedule, and any adverse effects before going home

DISCHARGE PLANNING AND LEARNING	• Blood thinner medication education by pharmacist
	• Ask questions to nurse concerning medications
	• Discuss stroke risk factors with nurse and physician
	• Discuss any sexual activity concerns with nurse or physician
		• Education on risk factors that cause stroke and signs/symptoms of stroke
		• MO Smoking help line 1-800-QUITNOW (1-800-784-8669)
		• Stroke Support groups and further resources
		  • Northland-Smithville Campus 816-932-6220
		  • American Heart Association 913-648-6727
		  • Strokes of Support 913-640-7555
		  • American Stroke Foundation 913-649-1776
		• Discuss ways to lower risk of future strokes
		• Discuss with physician when can drive and return to work
			• Understands to talk to physician if depression continues or worsens when discharged
			• Understands to discuss with physician if unable to control bladder
			
			Web site Resources:
			• Saint Luke's – Mid American Brain & Stroke Institute
			• American Stroke Foundation
			• American Stroke Association
			Free – Stroke Connection Magazine, call **1-888-4-STROKE**
			• National Stroke Association
			Free Stroke Smart Magazine, call 1(800) 787-6537
			• www.strokecenter.org

The suggested plan represents the initial desired course of treatment and goals of recovery. These are representative of average guidelines only. They should be reviewed periodically by the attending physician and other involved care providers. Deviations are generally expected and revisions to the plan should be made as warranted.

What Are the Risk Factors of Stroke?

The American Stroke Association has identified several factors that increase the risk of stroke. The more risk factors a person has, the greater the chance that he or she will have a stroke.

- **Increasing age** – The chance of having a stroke more than doubles for each decade of life after age 55. While stroke is common among the elderly, many people under 65 also have strokes.

- **Sex** – The latest data show that, overall, the incidence and prevalence of stroke are about equal for men and women. However, at all ages, more women than men die of stroke.

- **Heredity (family history) and race** – The chance of stroke is greater in people who have a family history of stroke. African Americans have a much higher risk of disability and death from a stroke than whites, in part because blacks have a greater incidence of high blood pressure, a major stroke risk factor.

- **Prior stroke** – The risk of stroke for someone who has already had one is many times that of a person who has not.

- **High blood pressure** – High blood pressure is the most important risk factor for stroke. In fact, stroke risk varies directly with blood pressure. Many people believe the effective treatment of high blood pressure is a key reason for the accelerated decline in the death rates for stroke.

- **Cigarette smoking** – In recent years, studies have shown cigarette smoking to be an important risk factor for stroke. The nicotine and carbon monoxide in cigarette smoke damage the cardiovascular system in many ways. The use of oral contraceptives combined with cigarette smoking greatly increases stroke risk.

- **Diabetes mellitus** – Diabetes is an independent risk factor for stroke and is strongly correlated with high blood pressure. While diabetes is treatable, having it increases a person's risk of stroke. People with diabetes often also have high cholesterol and are overweight, increasing their risk even more.

- **Obesity, elevated cholesterol, and elevated lipids** – Reducing your dietary intake of saturated fats and cholesterol may help reduce your risk of a stroke.

- **Carotid artery disease** – The carotid arteries in your neck supply blood to your brain. A carotid artery damaged by atherosclerosis (a fatty buildup of plaque in the artery wall) may become blocked by a blood clot, which may result in a stroke. If you have a diseased carotid artery, your healthcare provider may hear an abnormal sound in your neck, called a bruit (BROO ee), when listening with a stethoscope.

- **Heart disease** – People with heart problems have more than twice the risk of stroke as those whose hearts work normally. Atrial fibrillation (the rapid, uncoordinated beating of the heart's upper chambers) in particular raises the risk for stroke. Heart attack is also the major cause of death among stroke survivors.

- **Physical inactivity** – A sedentary lifestyle void of regular exercise can contribute to heart disease which may lead to stroke.

Saint Luke's Hospital
Kansas City, MO 64111

Clinical Path – Transient Ischemic Attacks

DRG _____   ICD9 _____   Anticipated LOS _____   Adm Date _____   Discharge Date _____

Medical diagnosis: _____

Physician: _____   Consultants: _____

_____

HEALTH RISK ASSESSMENT:

Do you smoke? YES NO	Previous Smoker	YES NO
Do you drink more than two alcoholic drinks per day?		YES NO
Do you exercise at least three times per week for 30 minutes or more?		YES NO
Do you have: Stroke warning signs or had a previous stroke		YES NO
High cholesterol		YES NO
Diabetes		YES NO
High blood pressure		YES NO
Heart disease		YES NO
Atrial fibrillation		YES NO
Migraine		YES NO
Family history (parents/siblings) of stroke		YES NO
Or heart disease		YES NO

Problem: **ALTERED CEREBRAL PERFUSION**   Modified: _____

Nursing Diagnosis: Altered Tissue Perfusion Cerebral   Resolved: _____

Generic Outcome Statement:

Initiated Date: _____

Expected Outcome: 1.   Patient will remain alert and oriented.
                                                  2.   Denies dizziness, sensory, or motor changes.

Nursing Assessment/   1.   Assess LOC, motor weakness, numbness, difficulty speaking, dizziness, vision changes, gait.

Intervention   2.   Instruct to call nurse if symptoms occur.

(Practice Standards)   3.   Instruct Pt/SO signs of TIA/Stroke.

Problem: **LEARNING NEEDS REGUARDING DISEASE PROCESS**   Modified: _____

Nursing Diagnosis: Knowledge deficit R/T Disease Process.   Resolved: _____

Generic Outcome Statement:

Initiated Date: _____

Expected Outcome: 1.   Patient will verbalize understanding of disease process and treatments.
                                                  2.   Patient verbalizes ways to modify health-related behaviors.

Nursing Assessment/   1.   Assess Pt/SO current knowledge.

Intervention   2.   Allow Pt/SO to verbalize concerns, questions, and frustrations.

(Practice Standards)   3.   Provide individualized instruction on specific aspect of care.
                                                  4.   Review, reinforce, modify teaching methods.
                                                  5.   Evaluate if Pt/SO can verbalize information taught.

Advance Directive [ ] YES [ ] NO ENACTED_____   CODE BLUE   [ ] YES [ ] NO

PATIENT IMPRINT   Date:_____   RN Signature:_____

SAINT LUKE'S HOSPITAL OF KANSAS CITY
Office of Clinical Practice Guidelines

The suggested plan represents the initial desired course of treatment and goals of recovery. These are representative or average guidelines only and should be reviewed periodically by the attending physician and other involved disciplines. Deviations are generally expected and revisions to the plan should be made as warranted.

	DATE: _____ DAY: ____1____	DATE: _____ DAY: ____2____	DATE: _____ DAY: ____3____
ASSESSMENTS	[ ] Allergy to iodine/dyes Yes/No [ ] [ ] Neuro assessment q2° x4 then q4° [ ] [ ] Vitals q2° x2 then q4° ____ Nuero assessment improving – no deterioration from baseline	[ ] [ ] Neuro assessment q4° [ ] [ ] Vitals q4° ____ Neuro assessment improving – no deterioration from baseline	[ ] [ ] Vitals q4° ____ Neuro assessment improving – no deterioration from baseline
CONSULT	[ ] Consult vascular surgery	[ ] Consult vascular surgery [ ] Consult dietitian for chol > 200	[ ] Patient discharged [ ] Scheduled for surgery convert to Carotid Endarterectomy Path
TESTS/LAB	[ ] SMA 18 [ ] Baseline PBG_____ [ ] Baseline O$_2$ sat____ [ ] EKG [ ] CT scan [ ] Carotid duplex study [ ] ECHO (TTE) [ ] Order Arteriogram [ ] Order TTE [ ] Call physician ECHO/Carotid duplex Arteriogram results	[ ] TEE [ ] Arteriogram post procedure checks [ ] Call physician ECHO/Carotid duplex Arteriogram results [ ] Call physician daily PT/PTT	[ ] Call physical daily PT/PTT
MEDICATIONS	[ ] [ ] Anti-coagulant_____ ____ PTT or PT therapeutic	[ ] [ ] Anti-coagulant_____ ____ PTT or PT therapeutic	[ ] Heparin Dc'd
TREATMENTS	[ ] [ ] Saline lock	[ ] [ ] Saline lock	[ ] DC saline lock
MOBILITY/ADLs	[ ] [ ] Bedrest ____ Participates in self care without symptoms ____ Tolerates up ad lib without symptoms	____ Participates in self care without symptoms ____ ____ Tolerates up ad lib without symptoms	____ Performs self care without symptoms ____ ____ Tolerates up ad lib without symptoms
NUTRITION	[ ] [ ] Low cholesterol, low fat, no salt added [ ] Order nutrition screening	[ ] [ ] Low cholesterol, low fat, no added salt diet [ ] Nutrition screening completed	[ ] Basic nutrition counseling completed
ELIMINATION	[ ] [ ] BRP	[ ] [ ] BRP	[ ] [ ] BRP
TEACHING AND DISCHARGE PLANNING	Explain pre/post procedure: [ ] Angiogram [ ] ECHO [ ] TEE – utilize instruction sheet [ ] Patient received path ____ Verbalizes understanding of patient teaching ____ Pt verbalizes understanding of pre-procedure teaching ____ Pt verbalizes understanding to notify nurse if any symptoms occur	[ ] Patient watches coumadin video [ ] Patient receives coumadin education material/tape [ ] Teach post procedure expectations following procedure (radiology post procedure sheet) ____ Pt verbalizes understanding of post procedure (radiology post procedure teaching) ____ Pt verbalizes own risk factors to future strokes (i.e. smoking, ↑ chol, afib, ↓ BP)	[ ] [ ] Review with PtAHA pamphlet – Facts about stroke – Warning signs of stroke ____ Pt verbalizes s/s of stroke ____ Pt verbalizes ways to modify life style to ↓ risk of stroke (stop smoking, low fat diet, exercise, BP control) ____ Pt verbalizes understanding medication education materials

[ ] = Interventions ____ = Expected Outcomes   **SYMBOL KEY:** "Initials" on a line means done and findings as expected
"✓" in a box means an intervention or item was completed
"o" in a box or on a line indicates the item was not pertinent to that shift
"*" in a box or on a line indicates the item was not done as expected

PATIENT IMPRINT   **SIGNATURE KEY:**

	DATE: _____ DAY: _____	DATE: _____ DAY: _____	DISCHARGE EXPECTED OUTCOMES DATE/INITIALS
ASSESSMENTS			_____ Verbalizes importance of notifying physician if symptoms re-occur
CONSULT			
TESTS/LAB			_____ Verbalized understanding need for any follow-up labs if ordered
MEDICATIONS			_____ Verbalizes understanding of discharge medications/ schedule and food drug intervention _____ Verbalizes importance of BP control
TREATMENTS			_____ Verbalizes available lifewise no smoke program if appropriate
MOBILITY/ADLs			_____ Verbalizes importance of exercise 3x's/week for 30 min _____ Verbalizes importance of 2 or fewer alcohol drinks/day
NUTRITION			_____ Verbalizes understanding of discharge diet/nutrition goals _____ Verbalizes ways to modify diet to ↓ risk of stroke
ELIMINATION			
TEACHING AND DISCHARGE PLANNING			_____ Verbalizes s/s of TIA _____ Verbalizes s/s of stroke _____ Verbalizes way to modify lifestyle

[ ] = Expected Outcomes
— = Interventions

SYMBOL KEY: "Initials" on a line means done and findings as expected
"✓" in a box means an intervention or item was completed
"o" in a box or on a line indicates the item was not pertinent to that shift
"*" in a box or on a line indicates the item was not done as expected

Time: _____
[ ] All nsg dg resolved
[ ] Valuables with pt
Mode: [ ] Wheelchair
      [ ] Stretcher
Accompanied by: _____
Discharge Nurse Initials: _____

PATIENT IMPRINT

SIGNATURE KEY:

___ _____   ___ _____
___ _____   ___ _____
___ _____   ___ _____

PHYSICIAN'S PLANS (ORDERS)

SAINT LUKE'S HOSPITAL
KANSAS CITY, MISSOURI

DATE	TIME	ANOTHER MEDICATION SIMILAR IN FORM AND ACTION MAY BE DISPENSED PER MEDICAL STAFF POLICY UNLESS CHECKED. ☐	"✓" Read Back Verification
		MABSI—Acute Ischemic Stroke Admission Orders	
		1. Admit as inpatient	
		2. Admit to Dr.	
		3. Diagnosis: _____ Ischemic Stroke _____ Hemorrhagic Stroke	
		4. Allergies:	
		5. Initiate Stroke Clinical Path	
		6. Diet:	
		_____ Keep patient NPO if patient demonstrates aspiration risk.	
		_____ Consult Communication Disorders to perform bedside swallow evaluation and give further	
		diagnostic or diet recommendations. Please order speech therapist's recommendations.	
		7. Weigh on admission and QOD.	
		8. Insert saline lock, flush every 8 hours and after usage.	
		9. IV fluids:	
		10. Discontinue Foley in 48 hours if patient's functional status allows	
		11. Use bladder scanner to assess for incontinence/retention. If PVR > 150 straight cath and	
		Reassess in 4 hours. Continue till PVR < 150	
		12. I & O	
		13. Telemetry for 72 hours then discontinue if no significant rhythm abnormalities.	
		14. Activity per clinical path.	
		• Bed rest and turn every 2 hours if hemodynamically unstable	
		• Day 2 mobilize including out of bed for meals and ambulation	
		15. Record on clinical path NIH Stroke Scale on admission and at discharge.	
		16. EKG upon admission if not done in ED.	
		17. Neurological assessment and vital signs per path.	
		a. Ischemic Stroke Parameters: If BP > 185 systolic or 110 diastolic on two readings 5–10	
		minutes apart notify physician for approval to use Acute BP Management Orders for	
		Ischemic Stroke.	
		18. Baseline PBG upon admission. If > 150 or patient known diabetic perform PBG QID and obtain	
		orders for glucose management.	
		19. O_2 saturation on admission and PRN. If sat < 90% place on O_2 at 2–4 L/min and titrate, notify	
		physician if unable to maintain O_2 sat > 95%.	

Affix Patient Label To **ALL** Pages (including Carbon Copies)

ALLERGIES / INTOLERANCES Height _____
Weight _____ ☐ kg ☐ lbs
Latex Allergy
Yes ☐ No ☐

PHYSICIAN'S PLANS (ORDERS)

SAINT LUKE'S HOSPITAL
KANSAS CITY, MISSOURI

DATE	TIME	ANOTHER MEDICATION SIMILAR IN FORM AND ACTION MAY BE DISPENSED PER MEDICAL STAFF POLICY UNLESS CHECKED. ☐	"✓" Read Back Verification
		MABSI—Acute Stroke Admission Orders	
		20. DVT Precautions: apply pneumatic cuffs while in bed.	
		21. Laboratory tests	
		a. Stroke Panel if not drawn in ED or transferring hospital	
		b. Fasting Lipid Profile next AM of admission	
		c. Hypercoagulability panel	
		d. Homocysteine plasma level	
		22. Physician Consultation	
		a. Consult Neurolgoy to assist with diagnostic workup	
		b. Rehabilitation Medicine Dr. Kelly/Steinle/Tait	
		c. Interventional Neuroradiology consult	
		23. Consult PT to evaluate and treat	
		24. Consult OT to evaluate and treat	
		25. Consult Speech therapy to evaluate for language/cognition disorder and treat	
		26. Consult dietary for nutrition evaluation	
		27. Diagnostics	
		_____ CT Head Scan Contrast _____ Y _____ N Indication: to follow-up stroke	
		_____ CTA Indication: evaluate cerebral arteries	
		_____ Carotid Duplex Scan Indication: evaluate carotid circulation (stenosis)	
		_____ Transthoracic Echocardiogram (TTE) Indication: embolic stroke source	
		_____ Transesophageal Echocardiogram (TEE) Indication: embolic stroke source	
		• Keep patient NPO after midnight prior to day test scheduled	
		• Educate on procedure and obtain consent from patient for TEE	
		• Discuss with cardiology need for antibiotic orders if patient has prosthetic valve	
		_____ MRI Head Indication: Localized infarction, small vessel disease	
		_____ MRA Head/Neck Extracranial Indication: evaluate extracranial circulation	
		_____ Cerebral Angiography Indication: evaluate Intracranial circulation	
		Other	

Affix Patient Label To **ALL** Pages (including Carbon Copies)

ALLERGIES / INTOLERANCES Height _____
Weight _____ ☐ kg ☐ lbs
Latex Allergy
Yes ☐ No ☐

PHYSICIAN'S PLANS (ORDERS)

SAINT LUKE'S HOSPITAL
KANSAS CITY, MISSOURI

DATE	TIME	ANOTHER MEDICATION SIMILAR IN FORM AND ACTION MAY BE DISPENSED PER MEDICAL STAFF POLICY UNLESS CHECKED. ☐	"✓" Read Back Verification
		MABSI—Acute Stroke Admission Orders	
		28. PRN Medications:	
		a. Laxative of choice (Milk of Magnesia 30 ml PO daily prn or fleets enema)	
		b. Tylenol 650 mg PO, elixir, or suppository every 4–6 hours PRN for temperature >100	
		29. Scheduled medications:	
		a. Docusate (Colace) 100 mg PO bid, capsule or liquid	
		Physician Signature:_____	

Affix Patient Label To **ALL** Pages (including Carbon Copies)

ALLERGIES / INTOLERANCES Height_____
Weight_____ ☐ kg ☐ lbs
Latex Allergy
Yes ☐ No ☐

PHYSICIAN'S PLANS (ORDERS)

SAINT LUKE'S HOSPITAL
KANSAS CITY, MISSOURI

DATE	TIME	ANOTHER MEDICATION SIMILAR IN FORM AND ACTION MAY BE DISPENSED PER MEDICAL STAFF POLICY UNLESS CHECKED. ☐	"✓" Read Back Verification
		MABSI—Transient Ischemic Attack Admission Orders	
		1. Admit as inpatient	
		2. Admit to Dr.	
		3. Diagnosis:	
		4. Allergies:	
		5. Diet:	
		6. Initiate and follow TIA Clinical Path.	
		7. Telemetry. Discontinue after 48 hours if no rhythm abnormalities	
		8. Neurological assessment and vital signs per path	
		a. Ischemic Stroke BP Parameters: if BP > 185 systolic or 110 diastolic on two readings 5–10	
		minutes apart notify physician for approval to use Acute BP Management Orders for	
		Ischemic Stroke.	
		9. Baseline PBG upon admission. If > 150 or patient known diabetic perform PBG QID and obtain	
		orders for glucose management	
		10. O_2 saturation on admission and PRN. If sat < 90% place on O_2 at 2–4 L/min and titrate, notify	
		physician if unable to maintain O_2 sat > 90%	
		11. Activity per path for extent of stay	
		12. Insert saline lock. Saline flush every 8 hours and after usage	
		13. IV fluid:	
		14. EKG upon admission if not done in Emergency Department	
		15. Diagnostic tests:	
		a. Fasting Lipid Profile next AM of admission	
		b.	
		c.	
		d.	
		e. Stroke Panel if not drawn in ED or transferring hospital	
		continued	

Affix Patient Label To **ALL** Pages (including Carbon Copies)

ALLERGIES / INTOLERANCES Height _____
Weight _____ ☐ kg ☐ lbs
Latex Allergy
Yes ☐ No ☐

PHYSICIAN'S PLANS (ORDERS)

SAINT LUKE'S HOSPITAL
KANSAS CITY, MISSOURI

DATE	TIME	ANOTHER MEDICATION SIMILAR IN FORM AND ACTION MAY BE DISPENSED PER MEDICAL STAFF POLICY UNLESS CHECKED. ☐	"✓" Read Back Verification
		MABSI-Stroke: Transient Ischemic Attack Admission Orders	
		15. Diagnostic tests continued	
		f. _____CT Scan of the head Contrast _____ Y _____ N Indication: to follow-up stroke	
		g. _____CTA Indication: evaluate cerebral arteries	
		h. _____Carotid Duplex Scan Indication: evaluate carotid circulation (stenosis)	
		i. _____Transthoracic Echocardiogram (TTE) Indication: embolic stroke source	
		j. _____Transesophageal Echocardiogram (TEE) Indication: embolic stroke source	
		• Keep patient NPO after midnight prior to day test scheduled	
		• Educate on procedure and obtain consent from patient for TEE	
		• Discuss with cardiology need for antibiotic orders if patient has prosthetic valve	
		k. _____MRI Indication: Localized infarction, small vessel disease	
		l. _____MRA Extracranial Indication: evaluate extracranial circulation	
		m. _____MRA Intracranial Indication: evaluate intracranial circulation	
		n. _____Cerebral Angiography Indication: evaluate intracranial circulation	
		o. Other	
		16. Physician consultation	
		a. Interventional Neuroradiology possible revascularization	
		_____consult and treat _____consult and confer only	
		b.	
		c.	
		17. Scheduled medications:	
		Physician Signature:_____	

Affix Patient Label To **ALL** Pages (including Carbon Copies)

ALLERGIES / INTOLERANCES   Height _____
Weight _____ ☐ kg ☐ lbs
Latex Allergy
Yes ☐ No ☐

II.   NIH Stroke Team Ischemic Pathway Summary   (NINDS, Aug 2004)

Assessment	Admission – 6 Hrs H & P, Baseline NIHSS	Hrs 6–24 Physical Assessment & NIHSS	Day 1 Physical Assessment & NIHSS	Days 2–3 Physical Assessment & NIHSS	Day 4 – Discharge Physical Assessment & NIHSS & MRS
	Evaluate Potential for Acute Therapies or Research Protocols				
Bed/Unit	ER or Stroke Unit, ICU if acute tx	Stroke Unit (ICU if acute tx)	→ → →	→ → →	→ → →
Vitals	Q15 min X 4 then q30 min X 4 then q 1 hr	Q 4 hrs	Q 6 hrs	→ → →	→ → →
Neurochecks	Q15 min X 4 then q30 min X 4 then q 1 hr	Q 4 hrs	Q 6 hrs	→ → →	→ → →
Cardiac Telemetry	Continuous	Continuous	As needed	→ → →	→ → →
Activity	Bedrest, HOB Flat	Advance as tolerated			
Diet	NPO until passes swallowing eval	Advance as tolerated	→ → →	→ → →	→ → →
Glucose	Accucheck q 6 hrs	D/C if normoglycemic	→ → →	→ → →	→ → →
	SSI prn	→ → →	→ → →	→ → →	→ → →
DVT Prophylaxis	SCDs & SQ heparin if nonambulatory	Continue prn immobility	→ → →	→ → →	→ → →
Nursing	Establish 2 18 g IVs	Maintain IV sites	→ → →	→ → →	→ → →
		Strict Is & Os daily	→ → →	→ → →	→ → →
		ROM Q 8 hs prn	→ → →	→ → →	→ → →
	Guaiac stool / record	→ → →	→ → →	→ → →	→ → →
	Daily weight	→ → →	→ → →	→ → →	→ → →
	Aspiration precautions	→ → →	→ → →	→ → →	→ → →
IV Fluids	0.9% NS @ 1–2 cc/kg/hr	D/C IVF if adequate PO intake	→ → →	→ → →	→ → →
Medications	Acetaminophen prn	→ → →	→ → →	→ → →	→ → →
	Ranitidine 150 mg IV/PO BID	→ → →	D/C unless ongoing indication	→ → →	→ → →
	Psylliium mucilloid 1 pkg PO BID	Continue as indicated	→ → →	→ → →	→ → →
	Docusate 100 mg PO BID	Continue as indicated	→ → →	→ → →	→ → →
	MOM or Dulcolax prn	Continue as indicated	→ → →	→ → →	→ → →
	Maalox Plus prn	Continue as indicated	→ → →	→ → →	→ → →
Rehabilitative Services	PT Eval Ordered	PT as needed	→ → →	→ → →	→ → →
	OT Eval Ordered	OT as needed	→ → →	→ → →	→ → →
	Swallow Eval Ordered	Swallow Tx as needed	→ → →	→ → →	→ → →
	Discharge Planning	→ → →	→ → →	→ → →	→ → →
Laboratory Tests	CBC/plts, PT/PTT, glu, lytes, BUN/Cr troponin, T&S, ESR, LFTs	PTT q 6 hrs until therapeutic if on anticoagulation	Daily CBC/pls, PTT, INR if on anticoagulation	→ → →	→ → →
		Additional W/U as indicated	→ → →	→ → →	→ → →
Neuroimaging	Stroke Protocol MRI or CT	Repeat for neurologic worsening	F/U Study if Received Recanalizaton Tx to R/O ICH	As indicated	→ → →
Other Diagnostics	EKG		TTE or TEE	Additional testing as indicated	
	CXR		Neck Vessel Imaging		
Secondary Prevention					
Antithrombotics	Initiate Per Protocol	Continue	Continue	Continue	Continue
Blood Pressure	Hold Unless SBP > 220 or per protocols	Hold Unless SBP > 220 or per protocols	Hold Unless SBP > 220 or per protocols	Initiate Per Protocol	Advance as tolerated
Statins	Initiate Per Protocol	Continue	→ → →	→ → →	→ → →
Education					
Smoking Cessation	Materials reviewed	→ → →	→ → →	→ → →	→ → →
Diet	Materials reviewed	→ → →	→ → →	→ → →	→ → →
Exercise	Materials reviewed	→ → →	→ → →	→ → →	→ → →
Stroke Warning Signs	Materials reviewed	→ → →	→ → →	→ → →	→ → →

STROKE DATABASE

There are several commercially available stroke databases, as previously mentioned (Chapter 2).

Some centers will want to develop a custom database. Included here is the Saint Luke's Stroke Database which might be a useful guide.

MABSI NEUROVASCULAR DATA COLLECTION SHEET

PATIENT NAME: _____ ADMISSION DATE: _____ DISCHARGE DATE: _____

MRN # _____ ACCOUNT NUMBER #: _____ SOCIAL SECURTIY #: _____ - ____ - _____

GENDER M/F   ETHNICITY _____   TELEPHONE: (____) ____-_____   DATE OF BIRTH: _____ AGE _____

ADMISSION DIAGNOSIS
- ☐ ISCHEMIC STROKE
- ☐ RETINAL ARTERY OCCLUSION
- ☐ HEMORRHAGIC STROKE
- ☐ TIA
- ☐ UNRUPTURED ANEURYSM/AVM
- ☐ CAROTID STENOSIS
- ☐ SUBDURAL HEMATOMA

☐ PATIENT TRANSFER FROM OTHER FACILITY

FACILITY NAME:
_____

☐ ENROLLED IN STUDY PROTOCOL

STUDY _____

PRIMARY CARE PHYSICIAN
NAME _____
ADDRESS _____
CITY, STATE ZIP _____
OFFICE PHONE _____
FAX NUMBER _____

MEDICAL HISTORY
(CHECK ALL THAT APPLY)
- ☐ **AFIB, HISTORY (427.31)**
- ☐ **AFIB DURING CURRENT ADMISSION**
- ☐ CAD'(41401, 412)
- ☐ DIABETES MELLITUS (250)
- ☐ DYSLIPIDEMIA (2720,2724)
- ☐ HEART FAILURE (CHF) (4280)
- ☐ VALVE PROSTHESIS (394, 395, 396)
- ☐ HYPERTENSION (401)
- ☐ PVD (4439)
- ☐ MIGRAINES (346.90)
- ☐ OBESITY
- ☐ RENAL INSUFFICIENCY (582, 584, 585)
- ☐ SLEEP APNEA (780.57)
- ☐ PREVIOUS STROKE/TIA/VBI
  - ☐ PRIOR TPA ADMINISTRATION
- ☐ SMOKER (CURRENT OR WITHIN PAST YEAR)
- ☐ ALCOHOL ABUSE
- ☐ DRUG ABUSE
- ☐ NONE OF THE ABOVE

PRINCIPAL PROCEDURES
(CHECK ALL THAT APPLY)
- ☐ ANGIOGRAPHY
  - ☐ EMERGENT
  - ☐ DIAGNOSTIC
  - ☐ ELECTIVE
- ☐ IV-t-PA
- ☐ IA t-PA (9910)
- ☐ IV-IA tAP
- ☐ RETRIEVAL DEVICE
- ☐ UROKINASE/PRO-UK
- ☐ ANGIOPLASTY (3950)
- ☐ STENT (3990)
- ☐ PFO CLOSURE (3552)
- ☐ ANEURYSM COILING (3881,3882,3972)
- ☐ ANEURYSM CLIPPING (3951,3952)
- ☐ ECIC BYPASS (3898)
- ☐ CAROTID ENDARTERECTOMY (3512)
- ☐ HEMICRANIECTOMY
- ☐ BURR HOLE
- ☐ STEREOTACTIC ASPIRATION
- ☐ AVM EMBOLIZATION
- ☐ VENTRICULOSTOMY
- ☐ ICP MONITOR

IN HOSPITAL COMPLICATIONS
(CHECK ALL THAT APPLY)
- ☐ ASPIRATION PNEUMONIA (5070)
- ☐ CLINICAL UTI (5990)
- ☐ DVT (453.8)
- ☐ PULMONARY EMBOLUS (415.19)
- ☐ INTRACRANIAL HEMORRHAGE
  - ☐ SIGNIFICANT
  - ☐ NOT SIGNIFICANT
  - ☐ LIFE THREATENING SYSTEMIC
- ☐ HEMORRHAGE
- ☐ SEIZURE
- ☐ HYDROCEPHALUS
- ☐ VASOSPASM
- ☐ NONE
- ☐ OTHER

MEDICATIONS AT TIME OF STROKE
(CHECK ALL THAT APPLY)
- ☐ ANTI-HYPERTENSION MEDS
- ☐ ANTICOAGULANT
- ☐ ANTIPLATELET _____
- ☐ DYSLIPIDEMIA MED
- ☐ DIABETIC ORAL/INSULIN
- ☐ NO MEDICATIONS

IN HOSPITAL CARE (CHECK ALL THAT APPLY)
- ☐ NEUROLOGIST OR NEUROSURGEON INVOLVED IN CARE DURING HOSPITALIZATION
- ☐ **REHAB ASSESSMENT WITHIN 24 HRS**
- ☐ **SCREENING FOR DYSPHAGIA IN STROKE PATIENTS**
  Date Screening performed: _____
- ☐ **DVT PROPHYLAXIS INITIATED BY 2nd HOSPITAL STAY** (FOR NON-AMBULATORY PATIENTS)
  Date/Time Initiated: _____
- ☐ **ANTITHROMBOTIC THERAPY WITHIN 48 HRS**
  Date/Time initiated: _____
- ☐ **Stroke Education Performed   Date:** _____

DISCHARGE DISPOSITION
- ☐ HOME SELF CARE
- ☐ EXPIRED
- ☐ HOME W/ HOME HEALTH
- ☐ DSG TO SLH REHAB
- ☐ TRANSFER TO SNF
- ☐ DSG OTHER REHAB
- ☐ TRANSFER TO OTHER HOSPITAL
- ☐ **HOSPICE/END OF LIFE CARE**
- ☐ OTHER _____

MECHANISM
- ☐ CARDIOEMBOLIC
  - ☐ PFO
  - ☐ A FIB
  - ☐ OTHER
- ☐ LARGE VESSEL ATHEROSCLEROTIC
  - ☐ MCA
  - ☐ BASILAR
  - ☐ ICA > 60%
  - ☐ CCA
  - ☐ OTHER (VERTEBRAL, ETC.)
- ☐ SMALL VESSEL OCCLUSIVE
- ☐ STROKE W/ NORMAL ARTERIES

- ☐ TANDEM LESION STROKE (ARTERY TO ARTERY EMBOLUS)
- ☐ VASCULITIS
- ☐ HYPERCOAGULABLE STATE
- ☐ OTHER IDENTIFIED CAUSE (AMYLOID HTN)
- ☐ HYPERTENSIVE HEMORRHAGE
- ☐ RUPTURED AVM
- ☐ RUPTURED ANEURYSM
- ☐ MECHANISM UNKNOWN
- ☐ TRAUMA/FALL
- ☐ DISSECTION (VERTEBRAL OR CAROTID)

ADMIT RHYTHM: _____
ADMIT BP ____ / ____ **T** ____ **P** ____ **R** ____
ADMIT GLUCOSE: _____
ADMIT: PROTIME/INR: _____
LIPID PROFILE: YES/NO DATE: _____
HOMOCYSTEINE LEVEL _____ ☐ ND
HBA1C _____ ☐ Not Drawn (ND)
ECHO - TTE: YES/NO   TEE: YES/NO

ISCHEMIC STROKE MANAGEMENT QUALITY STANDARDS OF CARE

NIH SCORING
ADM NIH_____   DISCHARGE NIH_____
□ NOT DOCUMENTED   □ NOT DOCUMENTED

STROKE ONSET: DATE/TIME_____
□ AWOKE W/ DEFICIT   □ ONSET UNKNOWN   □ TIME N/A

SLH ED TRIAGE: DATE/TIME _____   □ TIME N/A

DID PATIENT TRANSFER FROM OTHER FACILITY?
□ YES □ NO If yes, other facility triage **DATE/TIME:** _____

DATE/TIME INITIAL BRAIN IMAGING: _____ □ TIME N/A
□ TIME UNKNOWN

HT____'___"   WT_____ LB ____KG

IV T-PA STARTED IN? □ SLH ER   □ **OTHER FACILITY** □ NONE
(IF NONE, CHECK REASON WHY THROMBOLYTIC NOT CONSIDERED)

THROMBOLYTIC PATIENTS ONLY

DOSAGE: □ 0.6MG/KG □ 0.9 MG/KG

DATE/TIME IV THROMBOLYTIC ADMINISTERED_____

IV BOLUS DOSE_____MG   IV INFUSION DOSE_____MG

TOTAL IV DOSE_____ MG

SPECIAL PROCEDURES (FOR EMERGENT OR INTERVENTIONAL CASES)
Interventionalist: □ Grobelny   □ Akhtar
START DATE/TIME_____   □ ANGIOSEAL
                              □ PERCLOSE
PROC END DATE/TIME _____ □ VASOSEAL
                              □ SHEATH IN PLACE
FLURO TIME_____MIN   □ SHEATH REMOVED

CLOT FOUND? □ Yes □ no

INTERVENTION

□ **INTRA-ARTERIAL THROMBOLYTIC**

IA DOSE_____MG DATE/TIME IA INJECT: _____

□ **RETRIEVAL DEVICE**

PASSES_____   **DATE/TIME FIRST PASS**_____

TYPE DEVICE_____   retrieval successful □ yes □ no

ANGIOPLASTY/STENT
□ SINGLE □ MULTIPLE
□ RIGHT □ LEFT
□ INTERNAL CAROTID
  □ EXTRACRANIAL
  □ INTRACRANIAL
□ MCA
□ BASILAR
□ ACA
□ VERTEBRAL
□ PCA

% STENOSIS
□ < 50%
□ 50 – 70%
□ 70 – 90%
□ > 90%
□ 100%

□ SYMPTOMATIC
□ ASYMPTOMATIC

REASON THROMBOLYTIC NOT GIVEN
□ OUTSIDE WINDOW
□ DELAY IN ARRIVAL TIM
□ INR > 1.5
□ PROTIME > 15 SEC
□ CT SCAN FINDINGS
□ GLUCOSE < 50 > 400
□ BP > 185/110
□ PLATELETS < 100,000
□ NOT INCICATED

□ RAPID IMPROVEMENT
□ STROKE SEVERITY TOO MILD
□ SEIZURE AT ONSET
□ PATIENT/FAMILY REFUSAL
□ RECENT SURGERY, TUMOR, TRAUMA, STROKE, LP, ARTERIAL SITE, ACTIVE INTERNAL BLEEDING
□ OTHER_____

CLOT LOCATION

LEFT	PRE TIMI	POST TIMI
□ ICA AT ORIGIN		
□ ICA CERVICAL		
□ ICA PETROUS		
□ ICA CAVERNOUS		
□ SUPRACAVERNOUS		
□ ACA A1 SEGMENT		
□ ACA A2 SEGMENT		
□ MCA PROX M1		
□ MCA DIST M1		
□ MCA M2		
□ MCA M3, 4 MULTIPLE		
□ MCA M3, 4 SINGLE		
□ VA PROX TO PICA		
□ VA DIST TO PICA		
□ PCA P1		
□ PCA P2-P3		
□ L- RETINAL ARTERY		
RIGHT		
□ ICA AT ORIGIN		
□ ICA CERVICAL		
□ ICA PETROUS		
□ ICA CAVERNOUS		
□ SUPRACAVERNOUS		
□ ACA A1 SEGMENT		
□ ACA A2 SEGMENT		
□ MCA PROX M1		
□ MCA DIST M1		
□ MCA M2		
□ MCA M3, 4 MULTIPLE		
□ MCA M3, 4 SINGLE		
□ VA PROX TO PICA		
□ VA DIST TO PICA		
□ PCA P1		
□ PCA P2-P3		
□ R- RETINAL ARTERY		
□ BASILAR PROXIMAL		
□ BASILAR MID		
□ BASILAR DISTAL		

STROKE LOCATION
□ L HEMISPHERE
□ R HEMISPHERE
□ FRONTAL LOBE
□ PARIETAL LOBE
□ OCCIPITAL LOBE
□ TEMPORAL LOBE
□ SUBCORTICAL
□ INTERNAL CAPSULE
□ BASAL GANGLIA

□ THALAMIC
□ BRAINSTEM
□ CEREBELLAR
□ V-B DISTRIBUTION
□ SPINAL CORD

□ RIGHT □ LEFT
□ ACA
□ MCA
□ PCA
□ UNKNOWN

NORMAL ANGIOGRAM

TIMI RECANALIZATION
0 – no perfusion
1 – partial, minimal
2 – partial, incomplete
2IIa – partial < 50%
2IIb – partial > 50%
3 – complete
4 – not examined

TREATED AT A PRIMARY STROKE CENTER CERTIFIED DISEASE SPECIFIC CARE PROGRAM □ YES □ NO

SECONDARY PREVENTION

☐ **HYPERTENSION** ☐ TREATED ☐ NONE ☐ **DYSLIPIDEMIA** ☐ TREATED ☐ NONE ☐ CONTRAINDICATED ☐ **SMOKER** ☐ MED MGT CESSATION ☐ NON MED MGT CESSATION Date counseling:_____ ☐ **DIABETES** ☐ ORAL MEDICATION ☐ INSULIN	☐ **ANTICOAGULATION** ☐ TREATED ☐ NONE ☐ **ANTIPLATELET** ☐ TREATED ☐ CONTRAINDICATED ☐ NONE ☐ DIET INSTRUCTION ☐ **NONE**	**CONTRAINDICATION TO ANTIPLATELET/ANTICOAGULATION** ☐ HEMORRHAGE ☐ RISK OF BLEEDING ☐ REFUSED TX ☐ ALLERGY TO OR COMPLICATION R/T MEDICATION ☐ TERMINAL /COMFORT CARE DURING STAY OR AT DISCHARGE ☐ EXPIRED
		AT DISCHARGE FROM HOSPITAL: **WAS PATIENT IN AFIB AT DISCHARGE?** ☐ YES ☐ NO ☐ NA **WAS PATIENT DISCHARGED ON ANTICOAGULANT OR ANTI-PLATELET AGENT?** ☐ YES ☐ NO ☐ NA

ANEURYSM

HUNT-HESS GRADE ☐ 1 ASYMPTOMATIC ☐ 2 SEVERE HEADACHE; NO DEFICIT (EXCEPT CRANIAL NERVE PALSY) ☐ 3 DROWSY; MINIMAL NEURO DEFICIT ☐ 4 STUPOROUS; MOD TO SEVERE HEMIPARESIS ☐ 5 DEEP COMA; DECEREBRATE POSTURE	**ANEURSYM TYPE** ☐ FUSIFORM ☐ SACCULAR ☐ MYCOTIC ☐ TRAUMATIC	☐ SINGLE ☐ MULTIPLE TOTAL # ANEURYSMS TREATED _____

LOCATION		**ANEURYSM TREATMENT**	**COMPLICATIONS**	**COMPLICATION TREATMENT**
☐ RIGHT ☐LEFT ☐ BIFURCATION ☐ PARACLINOID ☐ PCOM ☐ ACOM/ACA ☐ MCA ☐ V-B	☐ PICA ☐ VB jxN ☐ BASILAR TRUNK ☐ TIP ☐ OTHER ☐ ANTERIOR ☐ POSTERIOR	DATE:_____ ☐ CLIPPING (3951) ☐ TRAPPING ☐ PROXIMAL OCCLUSION ☐ NEUROFORM STENT ☐ COILING (3881, 3882)	☐ HEMORRHAGE ☐ PRETREATMENT ☐ POST-TREATMENT ☐ STROKE ☐ DISSECTION ☐ VASOSPASM ☐ HYDROCEPHALUS ☐ INFECTION ☐ NONE	☐ VENTRICULOSTOMY ☐ SHUNT ☐ HHH THERAPY ☐ I A THROMBOLYTIC ☐ ANGIOPLASTY ☐ NONE
ANEURYSM SIZE ☐ SMALL/MEDIUM (< 13 MM) ☐ LARGE (13–24 MM) ☐ GIANT (> 24 MM)				

AVM

☐ AVM ☐ DURAL AVM **AVM SIZE** ☐ 1= <3 cm ☐ 2= 3–6 cm ☐ 3= > 6 cm **AVM LOCATION** ☐ 1=ELOQUENT ☐ 0=NON-ELOQUENT ☐ 0=DEEP	**VENOUS DRAINAGE** ☐ 0= SUPERFICIAL ☐ 1= DEEP ☐ VENOUS THROMBOSIS **SPETZLER & MARTIN SCORE** _____	**AVM TREATMENT** DATE:_____ ☐ SURGERY ☐ RADIOSURGERY ☐ EMBOLIZATION ☐ CLOT EVACUATION ☐ NO TX **COMPLICATIONS** ☐ HEMORRHAGE ☐ STROKE ☐ PERFUSION ☐ BREAKTHROUGH ☐ NONE	**AVM LOCATION** ☐ **RIGHT** ☐ **LEFT** ☐ FRONTAL ☐ FRONTAL ☐ TEMPORAL ☐ TEMPORAL ☐ OCCIPITAL ☐ OCCIPITAL ☐ PARIETAL ☐ PARIETAL ☐ CEREBELLAR ☐ CEREBELLAR ☐ BRAINSTEM ☐ SPINAL CORD ☐ MIDLINE ☐ OTHER_____

NURSING EDUCATION

Developing the critical thinking skills and clinical expertise of the nurses in the stroke center is a vital element in the success of the program. The content of three educational programs developed by the Saint Luke's Stroke Team is summarized here. These are presented twice a year.

Introduction to Central Nervous System and Peripheral Nervous System Anatomy and Assessment

- Two Dates in 2005 -
Wednesday, July 13, 2005
Tuesday, October 25, 2005

8:00 am – 4:00 pm
Saint Luke's Hospital

Mid America Brain and Stroke Institute

SAINT LUKE'S HEALTH SYSTEM

saintlukeshealthsystem.org

REGISTRATION FORM

Introduction to CNS & PNS Anatomy and Assessment

Name: _____

SS#: _____

Address: _____

Title: _____

Employer/Unit: _____

Daytime Phone: _____

_____ Please check here if you require any special accommodations. Someone from our office will contact you.

_____ July 13 – Spencer Auditorium
_____ October 25 – Peet Center Conf Rm

Course Fee:
_____ No Charge for SLHS Employees
_____ $ 50.00 fee for Community

Make check payable to "Saint Luke's Hospital" and mail to: Nursing Staff Development, Saint Luke's Hospital, 4401 Wornall Road, Kansas City, MO 64111

Introduction to CNS & PNS Anatomy and Assessment

PROGRAM OVERVIEW

This introductory presentation is designed to familiarize the nurse with neuroanatomy and neurological assessment. Content will focus on concepts and tools available for central nervous system (CNS) and peripheral nervous system (PNS) assessment. In-class practice and integration of theory will be provided through case study review and NIH Stroke Scale video scenarios.

Target audience is those nurses new to practice or new to neurological patient practice areas. This is an entry-level class.

PRE-CLASS GOALS

It is recommended that the participant prepare for this class by accomplishing the pre-class goals below.
1. Review CNS and PNS anatomy and physiology.
2. Review neurological assessment documentation.

OBJECTIVES

At the end of this course the participant will be able to:
1. Identify cerebral anatomical structures and their basic functions.
2. List tools available for performing a thorough nursing assessment of the CNS and PNS.
3. Utilizing the NIH Stroke Scale Assessment tool, correctly identify neurological deficits of patients pictured in video vignettes.
4. Through discussion of patient presentations, be able to differentiate location of neurological injury.
5. Describe the signs and symptoms seen with spinal cord injury in relation to the level of cord damage.

MORE INFORMATION

For more information, please call Nancy McEntee at 816/932-2111, or Ashley Peacock at 816/932-8603.

PLANNING COMMITTEE

Ashley Peacock, CES; Debbie Summers, APN Acute Neuroscience; Margaret Welch, APN Rehabilitation; Kay Carpenter, APN, Neurosurgery; Stacey Jett, Clinical Nurse, E1

AGENDA

Time	Session
0745-0800	Registration
0800-1000	CNS & PNS Anatomy and Physiology (With 10 minute break)
1000-1015	Break
1015-1145	Spine Anatomy, Physiology and Assessment
1145-1245	Lunch (On your own)
1245-1400	Assessment of the CNS
1400-1415	Break
1415-1545	NIH Stroke Scale
1545-1600	Wrap Up/Questions/Evaluation

PRESENTERS

Debbie Summers, RN, CS, M-SCNS, CCRN, CNRN

Margaret Welch, RN, CS, ANP, M-SCNS, CCRN, CNRN

Kay Carpenter, RN, MSN, CS-ANP, CCRN, CNRN

DATES AND LOCATIONS

This class will be offered two times in 2005.
Wednesday, July 13, 2005 – Spencer Auditorium
Tuesday, October 25, 2005 – Peet Center Conference Room

Class size on October 25 is limited to 24 participants. All employees must park in Employee Lots. Please allow extra time for parking and construction.

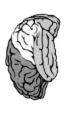

TO REGISTER

There are three ways to register for the class:
1) Complete the attached registration form and send to: Nursing Staff Development, Saint Luke's Hospital, 4401 Wornall Road, Kansas City, MO 64111. Non-employees of SLHS must include a $50.00 check made payable to "Saint Luke's Hospital".
2) Call 816/932-2111 and leave your name, the name and date of class you are enrolling in, and a call back number.
3) Send information via e-mail to nmcentee@saint-lukes.org

ACCREDITATION

Saint Luke's Hospital is an approved provider of continuing nursing education by the Missouri Nurses Association an accredited approver by the American Nurses Credentialing Center's Commission on Accreditation. This program is approved for 7.6 contact hours.

A $5.00 fee will be assessed to replace CE certificates.

NO SHOW POLICY

In order to make the most of our educational resources and as a professional courtesy to your colleagues—please call and cancel your enrollment as soon as possible. We understand that emergencies, illnesses and changes in work schedules occur. Call 816/932-2111 as soon as you know you are unable to attend—but no later than the start of the class. If you miss a class and have not cancelled in advance, you will receive a reminder notice that will be copied to your Manager. If you "no show" three times in a 12 month period, you will not be allowed to enroll in any additional classes for six months.

PROGRAM OVERVIEW

This intermediate level-class is designed to further the knowledge of the experienced Neurologic nurse in care of the acute stroke patient. The format will be mostly case scenarios analysis and dialogue that will be used to review etiology, pathophysiology, standard treatments, and recognition and prevention of complications.

Please review the pre-class goals for this course. This is not an entry-level course.

PRE-CLASS GOALS

It is recommended that the participant prepare for this class by accomplishing the pre-class goals below.

1. Clinical experience and basic understanding of the presentation and management of the Stroke patient.
2. Proficiency in neurological assessment, including use of the NIH Stroke Scale.

OBJECTIVES

At the end of this course the participant will be able to:

1. Review standard treatments for Stroke, including the physiologic effect that is the goal of each treatment.
2. Recognize risk factors, correlate neurological deficits of patient presentation to anatomical involvement, and anticipate plan of care for the stroke population.
3. Predict common complications found in the stroke patient population and describe ways to prevent and/or manage possible complications.
4. Discuss current research related to nursing care and patient outcomes.

Conversation in Care:
Intermediate Concepts in Care of the Acute Stroke Patient

AGENDA

1130-1200	Registration
1200-1330	SAH Case Studies
1330-1340	Break
1340-1440	Nursing Care and its Impact on Patient Outcomes
1440-1450	Break
1450-1550	Ischemic and Hemorrhagic Stroke Case Studies
1550-1600	Wrap-up/Questions/Evaluation

DATES AND LOCATIONS

This class will be offered two times in 2005.
Wednesday, March 16, 2005
Wednesday, November 16, 2005
Both classes will be held in the Spencer Boardroom

Class size is limited to 36 participants. All employees must park in Employee Lots. Please allow extra time for parking and construction.

PRESENTERS

Kay Carpenter, RN, MSN, CS-ANP, CCRN, CNRN
Debbie Summers, RN, CS, M-SCNS, CCRN, CNRN
Margaret Welch, RN, CS, ANP, M-SCNS, CCRN, CNRN

TO REGISTER

There are three ways to register for the class:

1) Complete the attached registration form and send to: Nursing Staff Development, Saint Luke's Hospital, 4401 Wornall Road, Kansas City, MO 64111. Be sure to mark which date you will attend.
2) Call 816/932-2111 and leave your name, the name and date of class you are enrolling in, and a call back number.
3) Send information via e-mail to nmcentee@saint-lukes.org

NO SHOW POLICY

In order to make the most of our educational resources and as a professional courtesy to your colleagues—please call and cancel your enrollment as soon as possible. We understand that emergencies, illnesses and changes in work schedules occur. Call 816/932-2111 as soon as you know you are unable to attend—but no later than the start of the class. If you miss a class and have not cancelled in advance, you will receive a reminder notice that will be copied to your Manager. If you "no show" three times in a 12 month period, you will not be allowed to enroll in any additional classes for six months.

ACCREDITATION

Saint Luke's Hospital is an approved provider of continuing nursing education by the Missouri Nurses Association an accredited approver by the American Nurses Credentialing Center's Commission on Accreditation. This program is approved for 4.4 contact hours. A $5.00 fee will be assessed to replace CE certificates.

PROGRAM OVERVIEW

This upper-level class is designed to challenge the experienced Neurologic Nurse in care of the acute stroke patient. The format will be mostly case scenarios analysis and dialogue that will be used to examine etiology; pathophysiology; cutting edge treatments; and recognition, treatment and prevention of complications.

Please review the pre-class goals for this course. This is not an entry-level class.

PRE-CLASS GOALS

It is recommended that the participant prepare for this class by accomplishing the pre-class goals below.

1. Clinical experience in management of the complex stroke patient.
2. Proficiency in neurological assessment, including use of the NIH Stroke Scale.

OBJECTIVES

At the end of this course the participant will be able to:

1. Discuss cutting edge research in, and treatments for, stroke, including the physiologic effect that is the goal of each treatment.
2. Recognize risk factors, correlate neurological deficits of patient presentation to anatomical involvement, and anticipate modifications to the plan of care for the complex stroke population.
3. Predict uncommon complications found in the vulnerable stroke patient population and describe ways to prevent and/or manage complications.

Conversation in Care: Advanced Concepts in Care of the Acute Stroke Patient

April 13, 2005
Auditorium
Helen F. Spencer Center for Education
Saint Luke's Hospital

AGENDA

1130-1200	Registration
1200-1330	Balloon Pumps and Perfusion Studies: A SAH Case Study
1330-1340	Break
1340-1440	Ischemic Stroke Case Studies
1440-1450	Break
1450-1550	Hemorrhagic Stroke Case Studies
1550-1600	Wrap-up/Questions/Evaluation

DATES AND LOCATIONS

The class will be held in the 2nd floor auditorium of the Helen F. Spencer Center for Education, Saint Luke's Hospital, 4400 Wornall Road, Kansas City, Missouri. Employees of SLH must park in Employee Lots. All others may park in the Broadway Medical Parking Garage at 4400 Broadway on the roof. Please allow extra time for parking and construction.

PRESENTERS

Kay Carpenter, RN, MSN, CS-ANP, CCRN, CNRN
Debbie Summers, RN, CS, M-SCNS, CCRN, CNRN
Margaret Welch, RN, CS, ANP, M-SCNS, CCRN, CNRN

TO REGISTER

Complete the attached registration form and send to: Nursing Staff Development, Saint Luke's Hospital, 4401 Wornall Road, Kansas City, MO 64111.

Employees of Saint Luke's Health System and employees of members of the Kansas City Stroke Education Consortium may attend the program for no charge.

The Kansas City Stroke Education Consortium membership includes:
American Stroke Association
Olathe Medical Center
Providence Medical Center
Research Medical Center
Saint Joseph Medical Center
Saint Luke's Hospital
Shawnee Mission Medical Center
University of Kansas Medical Center

NO SHOW POLICY

In order to make the most of our educational resources and as a professional courtesy to your colleagues—please call and cancel your enrollment as soon as possible. We understand that emergencies, illnesses and changes in work schedules occur. Call 816/932-2111 as soon as you know you are unable to attend—but no later than the start of the class.

ACCREDITATION

Saint Luke's Hospital is an approved provider of continuing nursing education by the Missouri Nurses Association an accredited approver by the American Nurses Credentialing Center's Commission on Accreditation. This program is approved for 4.4 contact hours. A $5.00 fee will be assessed to replace CE certificates.

Conversation in Care:
Advanced Concepts in Care of the Acute Stroke Patient

Wednesday, December 14, 2005

12:00 noon – 4:00 pm
Helen F. Spencer Center for Education
Spencer Board Room
Saint Luke's Hospital
Kansas City, Missouri

What is the Kansas City Stroke Education Consortium?

The Kansas City Stroke Education Consortium is composed of seven area hospitals and the American Stroke Association. These organizations have agreed to collaborate to enhance the educational opportunities for providers of stroke care at all levels of practice. Continuing educational credit will be provided by each sponsoring agency.

Education Consortium Goal:

The goal of this consortium is to provide evidenced based education emphasizing best nursing practices and patient outcomes.

Education Consortium Contacts

American Stroke Association
Judy James (913) 652-1917

Olathe Medical Center
Janiece Redwine (913) 791-3520

Providence Medical Center
Karen Highfill (913) 596-4627

Research Medical Center
Pam Smith (816) 276-3946

Saint Joseph Medical Center
Kathleen Henderson (816) 943-2400

Saint Luke's Hospital
Debbie Summers (816) 932-3777

Shawnee Mission Medical Center
Susan Stark (913) 676-2078

University of Kansas Medical Center
Jennifer Kieltyka (913) 588-0263

REGISTRATION FORM

Conversations in Care: Advanced Concepts in Care of the Acute Stroke Patient

April 13, 2005

PLEASE PRINT

Name _____

SS# _____

Address _____

_____

Title _____

Employer/Unit _____

Daytime Phone _____

_____ Please check here if you require any special accommodations. Someone from our office will contact you.

Mail to: Nursing Staff Development, Saint Luke's Hospital, 4401 Wornall Road, Kansas City, MO 64111

MORE INFORMATION

For more information, call Nancy McEntee at 816/932-2111 or Ashley Peacock at 816/932-8603

REFERENCE

1. California Acute Stroke Pilot Registry Investigators. The impact of standardized stroke orders on adherence to best practices. Neurology 2005; 65: 360–5.

Index